Rehabilitation of the Equine Athlete

Editors

MELISSA R. KING
ELIZABETH J. DAVIDSON

VETERINARY CLINICS OF NORTH AMERICA: EQUINE PRACTICE

www.vetequine.theclinics.com

Consulting Editor
THOMAS J. DIVERS

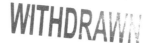

April 2016 • Volume 32 • Number 1

ELSEVIER

1600 John F. Kennedy Boulevard • Suite 1800 • Philadelphia, Pennsylvania, 19103-2899

http://www.vetequine.theclinics.com

**VETERINARY CLINICS OF NORTH AMERICA: EQUINE PRACTICE Volume 32, Number 1
April 2016 ISSN 0749-0739, ISBN-13: 978-0-323-41777-8**

Editor: Patrick Manley
Developmental Editor: Donald Mumford

Veterinary Clinics of North America: Equine Practice (ISSN 0749-0739) is published in April, August, and December by Elsevier Inc., 360 Park Avenue South, New York, NY 10010-1710. Business and Editorial Offices: 1600 John F. Kennedy Blvd., Suite 1800, Philadelphia, PA 19103-2899. Subscription prices are $270.00 per year (domestic individuals), $477.00 per year (domestic institutions), $100.00 per year (domestic students/residents), $315.00 per year (Canadian individuals), $601.00 per year (Canadian institutions), $365.00 per year (international individuals), $601.00 per year (international institutions), and $180.00 per year (international and Canadian students/residents). To receive student/resident rate, orders must be accompanied by name of affiliated institution, date of term, and the signature of program/residency coordinator on institution letterhead. Orders will be billed at individual rate until proof of status is received. Foreign air speed delivery is included in all *Clinics* subscription prices. All prices are subject to change without notice. **POSTMASTER:** Send address changes to *Veterinary Clinics of North America: Equine Practice*, 3251 Riverport Lane, Maryland Heights, MO 63043. Customer Service (orders, claims, online, change of address): Elsevier Health Sciences Division, Subscription **Customer Service, 3251 Riverport Lane, Maryland Heights, MO 63043. Tel: 1-800-654-2452 (U.S. and Canada); 314-447-8871 (outside U.S. and Canada). Fax: 314-447-8029. E-mail: journalscustomerservice-usa@elsevier.com (for print support);** E-mail: **journalsonlinesupport-usa@elsevier.com (for online support).**

Reprints. For copies of 100 or more of articles in this publication, please contact the Commercial Reprints Department, Elsevier Inc., 360 Park Avenue South, New York, NY 10010-1710. Tel.: 212-633-3874; Fax: 212-633-3820; E-mail: reprints@elsevier.com.

Veterinary Clinics of North America: Equine Practice is covered in *MEDLINE/PubMed (Index Medicus), Excerpta Medica, Current Contents/Agriculture, Biology and Environmental Sciences, and ISI.*

Contributors

CONSULTING EDITOR

THOMAS J. DIVERS, DVM
Diplomate, American College of Veterinary Internal Medicine; Diplomate, American College of Veterinary Emergency and Critical Care; Steffen Professor of Veterinary Medicine, Section Chief, Section of Large Animal Medicine, College of Veterinary Medicine, Cornell University, Ithaca, New York

EDITORS

MELISSA R. KING, DVM, PhD
Diplomate, American College of Veterinary Sports Medicine and Rehabilitation (Equine); Assistant Professor, Department of Clinical Sciences, College of Veterinary Medicine and Biomedical Sciences, Colorado State University, Fort Collins, Colorado

ELIZABETH J. DAVIDSON, DVM
Diplomate, American College of Veterinary Surgeons; Diplomate, American College of Veterinary Sports Medicine and Rehabilitation (Equine); Associate Professor in Sports Medicine, Department of Clinical Studies–New Bolton Center, School of Veterinary Medicine, University of Pennsylvania, Kennett Square, Pennsylvania

AUTHORS

HILARY M. CLAYTON, BVMS, PhD, MRCVS
Diplomate, American College of Veterinary Sports Medicine and Rehabilitation; Professor and McPhail Dressage Chair, Emerita, Michigan State University, East Lansing, Michigan; President, Sport Horse Science, LLC, Mason, Michigan

SUZANNE COTTRIALL, BA, BSc, MSc Vet Physio, MCSP, Cat A ACPAT
Co-ordinator PgDip, School of Veterinary Science, The University of Liverpool, Wirral, United Kingdom

JODIE DAGLISH, BVSc
Resident, Equine Sports Medicine and Rehabilitation, Department of Clinical Sciences, College of Veterinary Medicine and Biomedical Sciences, Colorado State University, Fort Collins, Colorado

ELIZABETH J. DAVIDSON, DVM
Diplomate, American College of Veterinary Surgeons; Diplomate, American of College Veterinary Sports Medicine and Rehabilitation (Equine); Associate Professor in Sports Medicine, Department of Clinical Studies–New Bolton Center, School of Veterinary Medicine, University of Pennsylvania, Kennett Square, Pennsylvania

DENNIS R. GEISER, DVM, CHT-V
Professor, Assistant Dean, Regenerative Medicine Section, Department of Large Animal Clinical Sciences, College of Veterinary Medicine, University of Tennessee, Knoxville, Tennessee

LESLEY GOFF, PhD, MAnimSt(AnimPhysio), MAppSc(ExSpSc), GDipManip, BAppSc(Physio)
Director, Active Animal Physiotherapy, Queensland, Australia; Lecturer, Equine Science, School of Agriculture and Food Sciences, Faculty of Science, University of Queensland, Queensland, Australia; Honorary Lecturer, Faculty of Health and Life Sciences, School of Veterinary Science, University of Liverpool, Liverpool, United Kingdom

KEVIN K. HAUSSLER, DVM, DC, PhD
Diplomate, American College of Veterinary Sports Medicine and Rehabilitation; Associate Professor, Department of Clinical Sciences, Gail Holmes Equine Orthopaedic Research Center, College of Veterinary Medicine and Biomedical Sciences, Colorado State University, Fort Collins, Colorado

KIMBERLY HENNEMAN, DVM
Animal Health Options, Park City, Utah

ANDRIS J. KANEPS, DVM, PhD
Diplomate, American College of Veterinary Surgeons; Diplomate, American College of Veterinary Sports Medicine and Rehabilitation; Owner, Kaneps Equine Sports Medicine and Surgery, LLC, Beverly, Massachusetts

MELISSA R. KING, DVM, PhD
Diplomate, American College of Veterinary Sports Medicine and Rehabilitation (Equine); Assistant Professor, Department of Clinical Sciences, College of Veterinary Medicine and Biomedical Sciences, Colorado State University, Fort Collins, Colorado

SARAH LE JEUNE, DVM
Department of Surgical and Radiological Sciences, University of California, Davis, California

COURTNEY LEWIS, DVM
Intern, Circle Oak Equine Sports Medicine, Petaluma, California

KHURSHEED R. MAMA, DVM
Diplomate and President, American College of Veterinary Anesthesia and Analgesia; Professor, Anesthesiology, Department of Clinical Sciences, College of Veterinary Medicine and Biomedical Sciences, Colorado State University, Fort Collins, Colorado

KEVIN MAY, DVM
El Cajon Valley Veterinary Hospital, El Cajon, California

CATHERINE M. McGOWAN, BVSc, MACVSc, DEIM, PhD, FHEA, MRCVS
Diplomate, European College of Equine Internal Medicine; Professor, Head of Equine Division and Director of Veterinary Postgraduate Education, Faculty of Health and Life Sciences, Institute of Ageing and Chronic Disease, The University of Liverpool, Wirral, United Kingdom

SYBILLE MOLLE, DVM, CERT, CKTIE
Private Practice, Viterbo, Italy

CARRIE SCHLACHTER, VMD
Diplomate, American College of Veterinary Sports Medicine and Rehabilitation; Medical Director and Owner, Circle Oak Equine Sports Medicine, Petaluma, California

Contents

Catherine M. McGowan and Suzanne Cottriall

> Physical therapy (physiotherapy, or PT) can be broadly defined as the restoration of movement and function and includes assessment, treatment, and rehabilitation. This review outlines the history, definition, and regulation of PT, followed by the core scientific principles of PT. Because musculoskeletal physiotherapy is the predominant subdiscipline in equine PT, encompassing poor performance, back pain syndromes, other musculoskeletal disorders, and some neuromuscular disorders, the sciences of functional biomechanics, neuromotor control, and the sensorimotor system in the spine, pelvis, and peripheral joints are reviewed. Equine PT also may involve PT assessment and treatment of riders.

Jodie Daglish and Khursheed R. Mama

> This article provides a brief overview of pain physiology and its relevance to equine patients. Objective and subjective techniques for assessing pain in the horse are described in depth. Pharmacologic and interventional pain modulation treatments are discussed with a focus on the rehabilitating horse.

Lesley Goff

> Physiotherapy assessment of the equine athlete is carried out by qualified physiotherapists, who use a functional approach to the assessment of the horse. Observation, clinical reasoning, good palpation skills and implementation of outcome measures are skills used by these professionals in their assessment of the horse. Equine physiotherapists attempt, where possible, to use an evidence-based approach to the assessment of the equine athlete.

Hilary M. Clayton

> The central body axis or core is a key component in controlling body posture and providing a stable platform for limb movements and generation of locomotor forces. Persistent dysfunction of the deep stabilizing muscles seems to be common in horses indicating a need for core training exercises to restore normal function. Core training should be performed throughout the horse's athletic career to maintain a healthy back and used therapeutically when back pain is identified. This article reviews

shock wave, and laser are discussed. Manipulative therapies, including stretching and use of core strengthening exercises and equipment, are outlined.

VETERINARY CLINICS OF NORTH AMERICA: EQUINE PRACTICE

THE CLINICS ARE NOW AVAILABLE ONLINE!
Access your subscription at:
www.theclinics.com

Preface

Innovations in Equine Physical Therapy and Rehabilitation

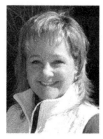 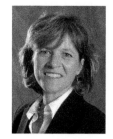

Melissa R. King, DVM, PhD   Elizabeth J. Davidson, DVM
Editors

It is with great pleasure that we introduce the first issue of *Veterinary Clinics of North America: Equine Practice* focused on equine physical therapy and rehabilitation. The goal of this issue is to expose the reader to the multiple facets involved in this ever-growing field. This is an exciting time as the science of equine rehabilitation is in its infancy. However, there are multiple individuals who have been working in the field of equine physical therapy and rehabilitation for decades, paving the way for others. This emerging area of expertise has expanded the team approach for the betterment of the equine athlete.

Equine sports medicine professionals have witnessed remarkable progress in the knowledge, skill, and maintenance of the equine athlete. Substantial advancements have been made in the fields of biomechanics, diagnostic imaging, regenerative medicine, farrier care, surgical procedures, and many others. Commonplace among our clients are the terms MRI, arthroscopy, and stem cells; with the availability of these sophisticated techniques comes an increased demand for enhanced function. This requires an allied professional team approach in order to maintain, restore, and improve movement, function, and activity. We hope to impress upon the reader that the art and science of equine rehabilitation is more than the latest gadgets, machines, and modalities but involves the ability to assess and manage a patient's global function. Clearly, the successful return to performance involves more than the pathoanatomical diagnosis.

We would like to thank the multiple authors who dedicated numerous hours of expertise to this issue. Each one of them is an expert in their field and has compiled

http://dx.doi.org/10.1016/j.cveq.2016.02.001
0749-0739/16/$ – see front matter © 2016 Published by Elsevier Inc.
vetequine.theclinics.com

the most up-to-date science available. This is an exciting time to be involved with such an innovative and rapidly growing field.

Melissa R. King, DVM, PhD
Department of Clinical Sciences
College of Veterinary Medicine
and Biomedical Sciences
Colorado State University
300 West Drake Street
Fort Collins, CO 80523, USA

Elizabeth J. Davidson, DVM
Department of Clinical Studies–New Bolton Center
School of Veterinary Medicine
University of Pennsylvania
New Bolton Center
382 West Street Road
Kennett Square, PA 19348, USA

E-mail addresses:
Melissa.king@colostate.edu (M.R. King)
ejdavid@vet.upenn.edu (E.J. Davidson)

Introduction to Equine Physical Therapy and Rehabilitation

Catherine M. McGowan, BVSc, MACVSc, DEIM, PhD, FHEA, MRCVS[a],*,
Suzanne Cottriall, BA, BSc, MSc Vet Physio, MCSP, Cat A ACPAT[b]

KEYWORDS

- Physiotherapy • Neuromotor control • Sensorimotor • Spine • Pelvis • Joints
- Horse-rider interaction • Veterinarian-physiotherapist team

KEY POINTS

- Physical therapy (physiotherapy, or PT) is an important allied health profession and can be broadly defined as the restoration of movement and function.
- Musculoskeletal PT is the predominant subdiscipline in equine PT, encompassing poor performance, back pain syndromes, other musculoskeletal disorders, and some neuromuscular disorders.
- Underpinning musculoskeletal PT are the sciences of functional biomechanics, neuromotor control, and the sensorimotor system in the spine, pelvis, and peripheral joints.
- Equine PT also, importantly, must involve the assessment of the rider and horse-rider interaction, as well as the tack and training aides used.
- Incorporating a veterinarian-PT team in the investigation, management, and rehabilitation of equine athletes adds a vital new dimension to equine sports medicine.

INTRODUCTION

Physiotherapy (called physical therapy in some countries) or PT is an important allied health profession whereby physiotherapists contribute an essential part to the care of individuals. The profession addresses a broad range of conditions in the young to the aged and from the severely debilitated to the elite athlete. Depending on the country, the legally protected title varies and includes physiotherapist, physical therapist, and chartered physiotherapist.

PT is an established, independent profession with an excellent reputation for evidence-based practice. Veterinarians have embraced PT and rehabilitation across

Disclosures: The authors have no conflicts of interest and nothing to disclose.
[a] Faculty of Health and Life Sciences, Institute of Ageing and Chronic Disease, The University of Liverpool, Leahurst Campus, Neston, Wirral CH64 7TE, UK; [b] School of Veterinary Science, The University of Liverpool, Leahurst Campus, Neston, Wirral CH64 7TE, UK
* Corresponding author.
E-mail address: cmcgowan@liverpool.ac.uk

the world, and the last decade has witnessed the development of a close working relationship between veterinarians and physiotherapists. The American College of Veterinary Sports Medicine and Rehabilitation is a specialist college wherein veterinarian diplomates have an excellent working knowledge of the benefits of working with PTs in a multidisciplinary team to care for the sports horse during competition and rehabilitation following injury or disease. Because most PTs in most countries need to work via veterinary referral and veterinarians and their clients understand and are demanding the unique skills base of a professional animal PT, the veterinarian-PT multidisciplinary team has become the gold standard in equine sports medicine and rehabilitation.

This review discusses the history and definition of PT (including animal PT) and the core principles of equine PT and its role in rehabilitation of horses.

HISTORY OF PHYSIOTHERAPY

PT is thought to have been practiced by physicians like Hippocrates and Galen from around the fifth century BC who advocated massage, manual therapy, and hydrotherapy to treat people.[1,2] In the subsequent centuries, the benefits of remedial exercise, hydrotherapy, and massage were known and practiced by relatively few. The earliest documented origins of PT as a scientifically based profession date back to Per Henrik Ling, "Father of Swedish Gymnastics," who founded the Royal Central Institute of Gymnastics in 1813 for massage, manipulation, and exercise.[2] In 1887, PTs were given official registration by Sweden's National Board of Health and Welfare.[3] Other countries soon followed, including Great Britain, which founded its first professional PT society in 1894 and was awarded its Royal Charter in 1920[4] (the Chartered Society of Physiotherapy), Australia in 1906, with the formation of The Australian Physiotherapy Association,[5] and the United States in 1917 following both an outbreak of poliomyelitis and the first world war and the subsequent need for rehabilitation.[6] The profession was established as The American Physical Therapy Association in 1921.

As PT has progressed, so has the database of information and journals specific to the area. The profession has its own PT evidence database (PEDro[7]) of more than 31,000 randomized trials, systematic reviews, and clinical practice guidelines in PT. Of relevance to animal PT is that much of the human research has been developed based on animal models, especially the cat (for example, spinal cord injury and rehabilitation models[8]), dog (for example, electrotherapies[9]), and pig (for example, back pain models[10]).

The profession is now represented internationally by the World Confederation for Physical Therapy (WCPT) that "believes every individual is entitled to the highest possible standard of care…underpinned by sound clinical reasoning and scientific evidence."[11] The WCPT currently has 12 internationally recognized subgroups: the Acupuncture Association of Physical Therapists; Association of Physical Therapists in Animal Practice (IAPTAP); Confederation of Cardiorespiratory Physical Therapists; Society for Electrophysical Agents in Physical Therapy; Federation of Orthopaedic Manipulative Physical Therapists; Organization of Physical Therapists in Mental Health; Neurological Physical Therapy Association; Association of Physical Therapists working with Older People; Organisation of Physical Therapists in Paediatrics; Private Physical Therapy Association; Federation of Sports Physical Therapy; and Organization of Physical Therapists in Women's Health.

World IAPTAP members include the following members:

- Animal Physiotherapy Group (Australia)
- Animal Rehabilitation Division (Canada)

- Finnish Association of Animal Physiotherapists (Finland)
- Fachkommission Tierphysiotherapie (Germany)
- Chartered Physiotherapists in Veterinary Practice (Ireland)
- South African Association of Physiotherapists in Animal Therapy (South Africa)
- Legitimerade Sjukgymnaster inom Veterinärmedicin (Sweden)
- Schweizerischer Verband für Tierphysiotherapie (Switzerland)
- Association of Chartered Physiotherapists in Animal Therapy (United Kingdom)
- Animal Rehabilitation Special Interest Group (United States)

DEFINITION OF PHYSIOTHERAPY

Encompassing the range of disciplines within the profession, PT can be broadly defined as the restoration of movement and function. PT involves using a professional assessment and reasoning process to select appropriate interventions or treatments for individual patients looking at physical, psychological, emotional, and social well-being.[12] The profession of PT uses an evidence-based, clinical reasoning process to underpin its management approaches.[13]

The clinical reasoning processes for PT are the same as those practiced by veterinarians, although the overall aim is different. The physiotherapist's aim is to reach a *functional* diagnosis, that is, identification of existing or potential impairments, activity limitations, participation restrictions, environmental influences or abilities/disabilities.[12] In contrast, the veterinary approach is usually to reach a *pathoanatomical* diagnosis (what pathologic processes are occurring and where they are located).[14]

Animal PT is an extension of evidence-based practice in the human field and is not merely the technical application of one or more treatment modalities (eg, massage, heat, cold, electrotherapy).[14] The difference in aims for PT is important because it dictates the treatment and rehabilitation options used. PT treatments are selected to manage sensory and motor disturbances and provocative factors in work or sport for functional improvement and activity-specific performance rehabilitation. Animal PTs use physical interventions, such as manual therapies, specific motor retraining, exercise prescription, and electrophysical agents, in conjunction with education and advice to restore function and quality of life.[14] Selection of the appropriate combination of techniques is based on clinical reasoning, assessment, and reassessment of the patient, with reassessment of improvement following treatment dictated by objective outcome measures.[14,15]

REGULATIONS AND THE TEAM APPROACH

The titles physiotherapist and physical therapist are protected by law in most countries and are regulated by its respective Act or equivalent and as such may only be used by individuals who are registered with the respective government body.

In some countries, PT or single modalities (eg, massage, hydrotherapy, Bowen therapy) are also practiced at a technical level by technicians. However, it is important that veterinarians understand the difference between technical and professional training, which is particularly the case in the those countries where referral to a physiotherapist by a veterinarian is required before PT is undertaken on animals, meaning the veterinarian is still professionally responsible for the animal throughout its treatment.

There are many advantages to using a professionally medically trained physiotherapist. The medical training allows PTs to have highly developed manual skills, based on their training with verbal feedback from their human patients. For many equine musculoskeletal disorders, there will also be an impact of the rider,[16] and the ability of the PT to professionally assess the rider as well as the horse cannot be underestimated. With the skills of clinical reasoning, evidence-based practice, and the ability to translate knowledge between species, the PT is an ideal partner in the veterinarian-PT relationship. Finally, the medically experienced PT is trained to work with and very often is the key facilitator of a multidisciplinary team that ensures the horse receives the most appropriate treatment. Within the equine environment, the multidisciplinary team predominantly consists of veterinarian, farrier, saddler, trainer, PT, and rider. The wider team can also include nutritionist, veterinary nurse, handler, owner, osteopath, and chiropractor. The professional PT is trained in being part of this team approach and understands the dynamics of these resources and how to make the best use of them in relation to their own clinical practice.

CORE PRINCIPLES OF EQUINE PHYSIOTHERAPY

As for the definition of PT, the core principles of equine PT revolve around clinical reasoning and evidence-based practice to inform assessment, treatment, and rehabilitation. During the course of rehabilitation, assessment and reassessment using objective outcomes measures are essential to direct progress and allow for modification of treatments[15] (See Lesley Goff: Physiotherapy Assessment for the Equine Athlete, in this issue, for PT assessment).

Musculoskeletal PT is the predominant subdiscipline in equine PT, encompassing poor performance, back pain syndromes, other musculoskeletal disorders, and some neuromuscular disorders. Underpinning musculoskeletal PT are the sciences of functional biomechanics, neuromotor control, and the sensorimotor system in joint function. Equine PT also, importantly, must involve the interaction of the rider and horse as well as the tack and training aides used. See Clayton HM: Core Training and Rehabilitation in Horses, in this issue, for a detailed review on functional biomechanics. So the focus in this section is on the principles of neuromotor control and the sensorimotor system in the spine, pelvis, and peripheral joints, and the horse-rider interaction.

Neuromotor Control and the Sensorimotor System

When training the equine athlete, the aims are to increase stamina, speed, and muscular strength as well as increase aerobic capacity, reduce the risk of musculoskeletal breakdown, and improve the biomechanical skill and neuromuscular coordination.[17] In order to do this successfully, the body coordinates several different systems. For the musculoskeletal system, these include soft tissue (muscle, tendon, ligaments, nerves, fascia), bone, and articular structures.

The basic functions of limb coordination, rhythm, and speed through all gaits is generated and controlled in part by central pattern generators (CPG). These specialized interneuron circuits located within the spinal cord have an ability to produce rhythmic patterned locomotion independent of supraspinal (brain) input.[18] There are separate control centers for the thoracic and pelvic limbs, although they are interconnected by long neurons to allow phasic coordination between the front and rear of the horse. Normal locomotion also depends on the ability of the central nervous system (CNS) to receive and process afferent sensory information (such as proprioceptive, visual, and vestibular input) from the sensorimotor system and to initiate and control movement in an effective, coordinated, energy-efficient fashion.[19,20] The relationship between neural and muscular (motor) control of movement is complex with reflexes (involuntary nervous system) as important as the voluntary activation patterns in control of spinal stability.[21] The final motor output during locomotion is a result of the CPGs and their modulation by an intact CNS.

The complex relationship between neural and muscular (motor) control of locomotion is referred to as neuromotor control.[22]

Neuromotor Control in the Spine and Pelvis (Axial Skeleton)

As well as modulating the dynamic limb patterns of locomotion, neuromotor control is highly important in providing a stabilizing core of muscles and their associated soft tissues to provide appropriate resistance to movement for a given joint. In the spine and pelvis, stability in humans has been clearly shown to be dependent on the contribution of 3 elements: (1) the passive structures (including the intervertebral disks, ligaments, joint capsules, and intervertebral joints); (2) the active structures (muscles); and (3) the control system (CNS), which exerts its effects on the muscles.[23] Spine equilibrium and stability, and resultant spinal function, are reliant on the coordination and control of muscle recruitment via neural input from the sensorimotor system.[20] A coordinated pattern of when and how the muscles activate, including neural feedback, compensatory mechanisms, and motor adaption to changing environments, are required. This includes neural feedback of changes in length and the rate of these changes in passive tissues and muscles, which trigger reflex muscle activity to counter the change and feed-forward control by motor cortex, whereby perturbations are predicted or anticipated and can be learned.[20,24]

The importance of these mechanisms in the muscular control of the lumbar spine and pelvis has been shown in a series of experiments in people whereby the transverse abdominus,[25] lumbar multifidus,[26] diaphragm,[27] and pelvic floor muscles[28] are all activated before and during perturbations created by rapid arm raises. This work demonstrated the predictable coordination of an array of muscles to provide a stabilizing core of muscles in the spine and pelvis in a manner primarily linked to the direction of reactive moments.[29] Such neuromotor control modulates muscular recruitment to fine tune the demands of internal and external forces, thereby ensuring appropriate motor responses to unexpected disturbances of movement and function.

Effective neuromotor control provides maintenance of functional stability, which is important in preventing excessive loading or movement that may lead to injury or degenerative changes or predispose to pain and dysfunction.[29] This stabilization is required to support the skeleton during locomotion and to ensure joints are maintained in their "neutral zone."[23] The neutral zone has been defined as the area of intervertebral motion where little resistance is offered by passive structures. It is a clinically important measure of joint stability in humans and has been shown to increase with degeneration or injury.[23] Unwarranted and unnecessary joint motion places the musculoskeletal system at risk of injury and is often termed "functional instability."[30]

Neuromotor control principles in physiotherapy (spine and pelvis)

The principles of neuromotor control have been successfully applied to humans with back pain. Research has shown that there is a reduced and delayed muscular recruitment and stabilization in patients with back pain, especially of the deep, core muscles of the spine and trunk.[25,31,32] Delayed muscle response times were also correlated with poorer postural control in patients with lower back pain.[33] This delayed onset of deep muscle activity does not reflect compromise of CNS performance caused by pain interference but has been suggested to be a result of adoption of an alternate postural strategy by the CNS, consistent with chronic adaptation to pain, and may serve to limit the amplitude and velocity of trunk excursions caused by limb movements.[34] However, pain adaptation may not be protective, and patients with back pain are at risk of reinjury because of a failure of protection of structures from overload and unwanted movement.[32] Similarly, in the low motion joints such as the sacroiliac joint in the pelvis, mild articular instability, or microinstability, may result in gradual remodeling of a joint.[30,35]

Knowledge gained from this research related to the changes in neuromotor control that occur with back pain has translated to the development of rehabilitation strategies based on motor control training approaches.[29] It is now universally accepted that clinical benefit can be gained if motor control can be changed to optimize the load and minimize unwanted joint motion on structures of the spine and pelvis.[29] Motor relearning strategies may focus on deep core muscles, such as the transverse abdominus and multifidus,[36,37] and may also involve targeting specific patterns of activation of muscle groups in combined functional movements, such as bracing the trunk,[38] to optimize motor control for spinal dynamic stability. There is evidence that this motor control approach can reduce low back pain intensity and functional disability, which is maintained following treatment.[36] Importantly, specific physiotherapeutic intervention in people with multifidus dysfunction following an episode of acute back pain reduced the rate of recurrence of injury to 30% in the PT intervention group compared with the controls, who had a recurrence rate of 84%.[37]

Similarly, knowledge of neuromotor control of the sacroiliac joint has been contributed to the ability of clinicians to diagnose sacroiliac dysfunction in humans. Noninvasive, manual tests have a high predictive odds ratio for sacroiliac dysfunction and are currently recommended over diagnostic joint analgesia.[39] These manual tests are described as pain provocation tests for the sacroiliac joint and are designed to compress the sacroiliac joint articular surfaces and/or stress the extra-articular structures of the joint. Manual tests are also used to assess the degree of movement and the quality of motion of the sacroiliac joint during application of manual force based on the amount of hypomobility/hypermobility, including analyzing movement of the sacrum relative to the pelvis in weight-bearing through the pelvis.[40]

Neuromotor control principles in equine physiotherapy (spine and pelvis)

Despite obvious limitations with respect to communication of specific exercises, the principles of neuromotor control have also been successfully applied in equine PT for the spine[41–43] and pelvis.[44] Stubbs and colleagues[41] applied the human model of researching the equine multifidus muscle to the horse and found striking similarities in structure and function. This research was used to develop and validate ultrasonography as a tool to detect reduced multifidus cross-sectional area associated with severe osseous abnormality in horses.[42] The use of this technique also enabled the identification of multifidus asymmetry in asymptomatic riding horses, which was improved by specific PT exercises over a 3-month period aimed at improvement of core muscle function.[43]

Diagnosis of equine sacroiliac disease using manual tests similar to that used in the human literature has been described[45] and is based on biomechanical and neuromotor control principles, including motion between the sacrum and ilium during the application of manual forces by a PT in vivo and in vitro.[44,46]

Neuromotor Control in the Appendicular Skeleton

As well as controlling muscular activity in the axial skeleton, neuromotor control and the sensorimotor system are important in controlling joint position and loading of the associated soft tissues in the appendicular skeleton. Fatigue[47] as well as injury[48,49] can alter the function of active elements (muscles) as well as sensorimotor inputs and neuromotor control, principally reflected in reduced joint position sense and proprioception. Furthermore, appropriate warm-up can improve joint position sense.[50]

Application in physiotherapy

Understanding neuromotor control and the sensorimotor system has informed treatment and rehabilitation of peripheral joint and soft tissue injuries, including the ankle,[51] knee,[52] and shoulder.[53] Proprioceptive retraining is an important part of rehabilitation, one example of which is taping. The aim of taping techniques is to stimulate mechanoreceptive and proprioceptive activity in the skin and superficial soft tissues (fascia, ligaments, and joints). Taping affects the sensory afferent activity from that region via stimulation of mechanoreceptors responding to skin stretch and compression during joint motion, improving sensorimotor afferent input, and ultimately, joint position sense.[54] Patellar taping was shown to improve control of the knee joint in both pain-free people with poor joint proprioception[55] and people with femoropatellar pain.[56] Similarly, the combined mechanical and proprioceptive benefits of taping for improving dynamic balance for preventing ankle sprains[57] as well as recurrence of sprains is well documented.[58] Taping, bracing, and manual therapy are used before exercise-based PT for an immediate effect on proprioception, whereas exercise-based therapies are used to maintain the improvements.[54]

Applications in equine physiotherapy

Taping has also been used clinically in horses for similar purposes. One study investigated the biomechanical effects of taping the fetlock in the forelimbs of horses, which showed an effect on fetlock flexion during swing and reduced peak vertical force during stance.[59] Although in this model, mechanical rather than sensorimotor effects were being investigated, the results suggested that changes seen may have reflected proprioceptive adaptations. More recent PT-led research has shown clear effects of tactile stimulation of the distal hindlimb in horses, causing increased hoof flight arc, increased peak flexion angles in the hindlimb, and increased concentric activity of the tarsal musculature.[60]

Horse Rider/Horse-Tack Interaction

In the past decade, there has been an emergence of research and growing awareness of the interaction between the horse, its tack, and the rider.[16] Riders have a large influence of horse's gait and can increase or decrease the expression of lameness detected by asymmetry.[61] Furthermore, this effect varies depending on the experience of the rider with the more experienced rider more likely to increase hindlimb lameness, presumably due to increasing collection and hindlimb usage.[61] Professional riders have been shown to be more stable than novice riders, with reduced motion detected by reduced vector angles between the rider's head and the rider's back and between the rider's back to the horse's head.[62] Experienced riders have also shown improved stability at the trot corresponding to more synchronous activation of the erector spinae and rectus abdominus muscles.[63]

Research into the effect of the saddle, in particular in the role of increased forces and "bridging" (where the weight of the rider is distributed on the caudal and cranial parts of the saddle but not throughout its lengths), has improved the understanding of saddle-induced pain.[64,65] Saddle slip has also been investigated. Despite previous assumptions about slip being due to a poorly fitting saddle or rider asymmetry, it has been shown that the saddle slip is most associated with hindlimb lameness or gait abnormalities.[66] Almost 53% of saddle slip was attributed to this and only 6% to rider asymmetry.[66]

However, in this study, rider asymmetry was present in 103 of 276 (37%) riders; even though most (78%) crooked riders did not induce saddle slip,[66] crooked riders may place additional stress on the horses' back, or indeed their own. It is already well known that elite athletes in many disciplines frequently show asymmetries, and the same is true of equestrian riders.[67] Less elite athletes or paralympic athletes may show more marked asymmetries that require extensive PT intervention.[68] Asymmetry can negatively affect performance in horses in various ways from the inappropriate delivery of aides to altered biomechanics of locomotion.[16,61] The important contact points of the rider and the horse are the lower limbs, pelvis, and, indirectly, the hands. Rider asymmetry, injury, or dysfunction can impact optimal delivery of aides and their interpretation by the horse. The relevance of the multidisciplinary team becomes significant here; the PT is well placed to identify rider asymmetry as well as assess and treat the rider and to ensure any suspected lameness is referred to a veterinarian and saddle problems are referred to a master saddler. Professional PTs are already highly trained in managing musculoskeletal disorders in the human athlete so the ability to assess the rider provides an important extension of the diagnostic workup. Furthermore, PT intervention can be an important part of the treatment and rehabilitation plan. Experienced riders after PT intervention to the pelvic region showed a marked improvement in symmetry compared with untreated controls.[69]

SUMMARY

In conclusion, PT is an important allied health profession that has been largely established following the wars and polio outbreaks that occurred at the beginning of the twentieth century. PT can be broadly defined as the restoration of movement and function. There are many subdisciplines of PT, but musculoskeletal PT is the predominant subdiscipline in equine PT, encompassing poor performance, back pain syndromes, other musculoskeletal disorders, and some neuromuscular disorders. Underpinning musculoskeletal PT are the sciences of functional biomechanics, neuromotor control, and the sensorimotor system in the spine, pelvis, and peripheral joints. Equine PT also, importantly, must involve the rider and horse-rider interaction as well as the tack and training aides used. Incorporating a veterinarian-physiotherapist team in the investigation, management, and rehabilitation of equine athletes adds a vital new dimension to equine sports medicine.

REFERENCES

1. Pettman E. A history of manipulative therapy. J Man Manip Ther 2007;15:165–74.
2. Kumar PS. Thinking out of the box. Int J Physiother Rehabil 2010;1:01–4.
3. Swedish National Board of Health and Welfare. 2007. Available at: www.socialstyrelsen.se/english. Accessed February 2007.
4. Anonymous, CSP history, The Chartered Society of Physiotherapy. Available at: www.csp.org.uk. Accessed October 8, 2015.
5. Anonymous, History, the Australian Physiotherapy Association. Available at: www.physiotherapy.asn.au. Accessed October 8, 2015.
6. American Physical Therapy Association history of the profession of physical therapy. In: Today's physical therapist: a comprehensive review of a 21st-century health care profession. 2011. p. 6–9.
7. Available at: http://www.pedro.org.au/. Accessed October 8, 2015.
8. Cohen-Adad J, Martinez M, Delivet-Mongrain H, et al. Recovery of locomotion after partial spinal cord lesions in cats: assessment using behavioral, electrophysiological and imaging techniques. Acta Neurobiol Exp (Wars) 2014;74:142–57.
9. Gu XQ, Li YM, Guo J, et al. Effect of low intensity pulsed ultrasound on repairing the periodontal bone of Beagle canines. Asian Pac J Trop Med 2014;7:325–8.

10. Hodges P, Holm AK, Hansson T, et al. Rapid atrophy of the lumbar multifidus follows experimental disc or nerve root injury. Spine (Phila Pa 1976) 2006;31: 2926–33.
11. Anonymous. World Confederation for Physical Therapy. 2015. Available at: http:// www.wcpt.org/. Accessed October 8, 2015.
12. World Confederation for Physical Therapy (2011) Policy Statement: description of physical therapy, World Confederation for Physical Therapy. Available at: www. wcpt.org/policy/ps-descriptionPT. Accessed October 8, 2015.
13. Hanekom S, Gosselink R, Dean E, et al. The development of a clinical management algorithm for early physical activity and mobilization of critically ill patients: synthesis of evidence and expert opinion and its translation into practice. Clin Rehabil 2011;25(9):771–87.
14. McGowan CM, Stubbs NC, Jull GA. Equine physiotherapy: a comparative view of the science underlying the profession. Equine Vet J 2007;39(1):90–4.
15. Goff L. Physiotherapy assessment for animals. In: McGowan CM, Goff L, editors. Animal physiotherapy. Second Edition, Wiley-Blackwell, West Sussex UK. Chapter 11, 2016. p. 171–96.
16. Greve L, Dyson S. The horse-saddle-rider interaction. Vet J 2013;195(3):275–81.
17. Marlin D, Nankervis KJ. Equine exercise physiology. Oxford, UK: John Wiley & Sons; 2013.
18. Golubitsky M, Stewart I, Buono PL, et al. Symmetry in locomotor central pattern generators and animal gaits. Nature 1999;401(6754):693–5.
19. Lam T, Anderschitz M, Dietz V. Contribution of feedback and feedforward strategies to locomotor adaptations. J Neurophysiol 2006;95(2):766–73.
20. van Dieën JH, Kingma I. Spine function and low back pain: interactions of active and passive structures. In: Hodges PW, Cholewicki J, van Dieën JH, editors. Spinal control: the rehabilitation of back pain: state of the art and science. Edinburgh, UK: Churchill Livingstone-Elsevier; 2013. p. 41–57.
21. Moorhouse KM, Granata KP. Role of reflex dynamics in spinal stability: intrinsic muscle stiffness alone is insufficient for stability. J Biomech 2007;40:1058–65.
22. Gregory B. The biomechanics of equine locomotion. In: Hodgson DR, McKeever K, McGowan CM, editors. The athletic horse: principles and practice of equine sports medicine. 2nd edition. St. Louis: Elsevier/Saunders; 2013. p. 282–93.
23. Panjabi MM. The stabilizing system of the spine. Part I. Function, dysfunction, adaptation, and enhancement. J Spinal Disord 1992;5:383–9.
24. Reeves NP, Cholewicki J, Pearcy M, et al. How can models of motor control be useful for understanding low back pain? In: Hodges PW, Cholewicki J, van Dieën JH, editors. Spinal control: the rehabilitation of back pain: state of the art and science. Edinburgh, UK: Churchill Livingstone-Elsevier; 2013. p. 187–93.
25. Hodges PW, Richardson CA. Inefficient muscular stabilization of the lumbar spine associated with low back pain. A motor control evaluation of transversus abdominis. Spine (Phila Pa 1976) 1996;21:2640–50.
26. Moseley GL, Hodges PW, Gandevia SC. Deep and superficial fibers of lumbar multifidus are differentially active during voluntary arm movements. Spine 2002; 27:E29–36, 24.
27. Hodges PW, Butler JE, McKenzie D, et al. Contraction of the human diaphragm during postural adjustments. J Physiol 1997;505:239–48.
28. Hodges PW, Sapsford R, Pengel LHM. Postural and respiratory functions of the pelvic floor muscles. Neurourol Urodyn 2007;26:362–71.

29. Hodges PW, McGill S, Hides JA. Motor control of the spine and changes in pain: debate about the extrapolation from research observations of motor control strategies to effective treatments for back pain. In: Hodges PW, Cholewicki J, van Dieën JH, editors. Spinal control: the rehabilitation of back pain: state of the art and science. Edinburgh, UK: Churchill Livingstone-Elsevier; 2013.

30. Goff LM, Jeffcott LB, Jasiewicz J, et al. Structural and biomechanical aspects of equine sacroiliac joint function and their relationship to clinical disease. Vet J 2008;176(3):281–93.

31. Hodges PW, Richardson CA. Altered trunk muscle recruitment in people with low back pain with upper limb movement at different speeds. Arch Phys Med Rehabil 1999;80(9):1005–12.

32. MacDonald D, Moseley GL, Hodges PW. Why do some patients keep hurting their back? Evidence of ongoing back muscle dysfunction during remission from recurrent back pain. Pain 2009;142(3):183–8.

33. Radebold A, Cholewicki J, Polzhofer GK, et al. Impaired postural control of the lumbar spine is associated with delayed muscle response times in patients with chronic idiopathic low back pain. Spine 2001;26:724–30.

34. Moseley GL, Hodges PW. Are the changes in postural control associated with low back pain caused by pain interference? Clin J Pain 2005;21(4):323–9.

35. Brolinson P, Kozar A, Cibor G. Sacroiliac joint dysfunction in athletes. Curr Sports Med Rep 2003;2:47–56.

36. O'Sullivan PB, Twomey LT, Allison GT. Evaluation of specific stabilizing exercise in the treatment of chronic low back pain with radiologic diagnosis of spondylolysis or spondylolisthesis. Spine 1997;22:2959.

37. Hides JA, Jull GA, Richardson CA. Long-term effects of specific stabilizing exercises for first-episode low back pain. Spine 2001;26:243–8.

38. Grenier SG, McGill SM. Quantification of lumbar stability by using 2 different abdominal activation strategies. Arch Phys Med Rehabil 2007;88(1):54–62.

39. Szadek KM, van der Wurff P, van Tulder MW, et al. Diagnostic validity of criteria for sacroiliac joint pain: a systematic review. J Pain 2009;10(4):354–68.

40. Lee D. The pelvic girdle—an approach to the examination and treatment of the lumbo-pelvic-hip region. 3rd edition. Edinburgh, UK: Churchill Livingstone Elsevier; 2004. ix.

41. Stubbs NC, Hodges PW, Jeffcott LB, et al. Functional anatomy of the caudal thoracolumbar and lumbosacral spine in the horse. Equine Vet J Suppl 2006;(36): 393–9.

42. Stubbs NC, Riggs CM, Hodges PW, et al. Osseous spinal pathology and epaxial muscle ultrasonography in Thoroughbred racehorses. Equine Vet J Suppl 2010;(38):654–61.

43. Stubbs NC, Kaiser LJ, Hauptman J, et al. Dynamic mobilisation exercises increase cross sectional area of musculus multifidus. Equine Vet J 2011;43(5): 522–9.

44. Goff LM, Jasiewicz J, Jeffcott LB, et al. Movement between the equine ilium and sacrum: in vivo and in vitro studies. Equine Vet J Suppl 2006;(36):457–61.

45. Varcoe-Cocks K, Sagar KN, Jeffcott LB, et al. Pressure algometry to quantify muscle pain in racehorses with suspected sacroiliac dysfunction. Equine Vet J 2006;38:558–62.

46. Goff L, Van Weeren PR, Jeffcott L, et al. Quantification of equine sacral and iliac motion during gait: a comparison between motion capture with skin-mounted and bone-fixated sensors. Equine Vet J Suppl 2010;(38):468–74.

47. Mohammadi F, Azma K, Naseh I, et al. Military exercises, knee and ankle joint position sense, and injury in male conscripts: a pilot study. J Athl Train 2013;48(6): 790–6.
48. Cronström A, Ageberg E. Association between sensory function and mediolateral knee position during functional tasks in patients with anterior cruciate ligament injury. BMC Musculoskelet Disord 2014;13(15):430.
49. Franettovich Smith MM, Honeywill C, Wyndow N, et al. Neuromotor control of gluteal muscles in runners with Achilles tendinopathy. Med Sci Sports Exerc 2014;46(3):594–9.
50. Salgado E, Ribeiro F, Oliveira J. Joint-position sense is altered by football pre-participation warm-up exercise and match induced fatigue. Knee 2015;22(3): 243–8.
51. Munn J, Sullivan SJ, Schneiders AG. Evidence of sensorimotor deficits in functional ankle instability: a systematic review with meta-analysis. J Sci Med Sport 2010;13(1):2–12.
52. Kvist J. Rehabilitation following anterior cruciate ligament injury. Sports Med 2004;34(4):269–80.
53. Myers JB, Wassinger CA, Lephart SM. Sensorimotor contribution to shoulder stability: effect of injury and rehabilitation. Man Ther 2006;11:197.
54. Clark NC, Röijezon U, Treleaven J. Proprioception in musculoskeletal rehabilitation. Part 2: clinical assessment and intervention. Man Ther 2015;20(3):378–87.
55. Callaghan MJ, Selfe J, Bagley PJ, et al. The effects of patellar taping on knee joint proprioception. J Athl Train 2002;37:19.
56. Herrington L. The effect of corrective taping of the patella on patella position as defined by MRI. Res Sports Med 2006;14:215.
57. Lee BG, Lee JH. Immediate effects of ankle balance taping with kinesiology tape on the dynamic balance of young players with functional ankle instability. Technol Health Care 2015;23(3):333–41.
58. Kemler E, van de Port I, Schmikli S, et al. Effects of soft bracing or taping on a lateral ankle sprain: a non-randomised controlled trial evaluating recurrence rates and residual symptoms at one year. J Foot Ankle Res 2015;8:13.
59. Ramón T, Prades M, Armengou L, et al. Effects of athletic taping of the fetlock on distal limb mechanics. Equine Vet J 2004;36:764–8.
60. Clayton HM, White AD, Kaiser LJ, et al. Hindlimb response to tactile stimulation of the pastern and coronet. Equine Vet J 2010;42:227–33.
61. Licka T, Kapaun M, Peham C. Influence of rider on lameness in trotting horses. Equine Vet J 2004;36(8):734–6.
62. Peham C, Licka T, Kapaun M, et al. A new method to quantify harmony of the horse–rider system in dressage. Sports Eng 2001;4:95–101.
63. Terada K. Comparison of head movement and EMG activity of muscles between advanced and novice horseback riders at different gaits. J Equine Sci 2000; 11(4):83–90.
64. Harman JC. Practical use of a computerized saddle pressure measuring device to determine the effects of saddle pads on the horse's back. J Equine Vet Sci 1994;14:606.
65. von Peinen K, Wiestner T, von Rechenberg B, et al. Relationship between saddle pressure measurements and clinical signs of saddle soreness at the withers. Equine Vet J 2010;42(Suppl 38):650–3.
66. Greve L, Dyson SJ. The interrelationship of lameness, saddle slip and back shape in the general sports horse population. Equine Vet J 2014;46(6):687–94.

67. Symes D, Ellis R. A preliminary study into rider asymmetry within equitation. Vet J 2009;181(1):34–7.
68. Athanasopoulos S, Mandalidis D, Tsakoniti A, et al. The 2004 paralympic games: physiotherapy services in the paralympic village polyclinic. Open Sports Med J 2009;3:1–8.
69. Nevison CM, Timmis MA. The effect of physiotherapy intervention to the pelvic region of experienced riders on seated postural stability and the symmetry of pressure distribution to the saddle: a preliminary study. J Vet Behav Clin Appl Res 2013;8(4):261–4.

Pain

Its Diagnosis and Management in the Rehabilitation of Horses

Jodie Daglish, BVSc[a], Khursheed R. Mama, DVM[b],*

KEYWORDS

- Equine • Pain • Analgesia • Musculoskeletal • Rehabilitation
- Interventional therapy

KEY POINTS

- Pain recognition in the horse is assisted by use of evolving observational and objective measures, including composite pain scales and gait analysis technology.
- Pain modulation may be provided to the horse using pharmacologic, manual, and interventional therapies.
- Pain recognition, modulation and consistent monitoring may help to provide specifically tailored rehabilitation programmes that can optimize return to athletic function.

INTRODUCTION

Assessment of acute or chronic injury must include determination of pain related to tissue damage to facilitate development of an appropriate treatment and rehabilitation plan. The International Association for the Study of Pain defines pain as an unpleasant sensory and emotional experience associated with actual or potential tissue damage or described in terms of such damage.[1] Assessing pain in the horse is complex and dynamic, and techniques regularly used to assess pain in humans and other species do not readily transfer to the horse.[2,3] Recent interest has resulted in increasing knowledge and availability of objective measures for pain evaluation in horses.[4–8] Following a brief review of pain physiology, the focus of this article is on the tools available for the diagnosis and management of musculoskeletal pain and their consideration in developing rehabilitation protocols.

Disclosure statement: The authors have nothing to disclose.
[a] Equine Sports Medicine and Rehabilitation, Department of Clinical Sciences, College of Veterinary Medicine and Biomedical Sciences, Colorado State University, 300 West Drake Road, Fort Collins, CO 80523, USA; [b] Veterinary, Anesthesiology, Department of Clinical Sciences, College of Veterinary Medicine and Biomedical Sciences, Colorado State University, Fort Collins, CO 80523, USA
* Corresponding author.
E-mail address: kmama@colostate.edu

BRIEF REVIEW OF PAIN PHYSIOLOGY

The perception of pain is highly complex and multifaceted, relying on differential processing of noxious stimuli by specialized neural pathways depending on the type and intensity of signal.

- Nociceptors are sensory receptors that transduce and encode signals in response to noxious stimuli from chemical, thermal, and mechanical sources.[9]
- Nociceptive stimulation triggers action potentials within high-threshold afferent neurons (unmyelinated C-fibers or weakly myelinated Aδ-fibers) whose cell bodies are located in the dorsal root ganglia.[10]
- Nociceptive stimuli are projected through central pain signaling neurons in the spinal cord to the higher brain centers where pain is perceived by the animal.
- Excitatory glutamate receptors and inhibitory GABAergic and glycinergic receptors[11] are considered the primary dorsal horn nociceptive pathway neuropeptides.
- Transmission of nociceptive signals from the peripheral nerve through the spinal cord is subject to modulation by alternate input, intrinsic neurons, and controls emanating from the brain. For example, nociceptive input can be modulated by increasing afferent input from nonpainful stimulus (eg, rubbing area of wound following touching a hot stove).[12]
- In people the somatosensory cortices are associated with sensory pain perception, and the cerebellum is involved in the processing of responses to noxious stimulation.[13,14]
- Descending neural pathways are broadly considered inhibitory and are modulated by concentrations of endogenous opioids, cholecystokinin, neurotensin, acetylcholine, cannabinoids, α_2-adrenergic agonists, and serotonin, propagating inhibitory signals from the higher centers to the peripheral tissues.[15]
- Local and neural effects at the site of injury result in upregulation of vasoactive compounds and neuropeptides.[10] These compounds and neuropeptides, in turn, stimulate epidermal and immune cells, leading to vasodilation, plasma extravasation, and smooth muscle contraction.

Although the complexity and plasticity of the pain pathway provides challenges in pain recognition, advances in diagnostic technologies and knowledge of targets for therapeutic modulation have improved our capacity to provide pain relief. Treatment approaches are likely to differ further depending on the nature of the pain state, which broadly may be categorized as acute or chronic.

Acute Pain

This pain generally follows injury wherein the withdrawal from noxious stimulus alone fails to prevent tissue damage and results in activation of the afferent nociceptive pathway.[10] The response generated by the body is intended to facilitate removal of injured or damaged cells, eliminate foreign material, minimize further damage, and provide an environment for tissue regeneration. Heat, swelling, redness, and loss of function are caused by actions of chemical substances (eg, bradykinin, cytokines, prostaglandins), result in inflammatory pain and may cause primary hyperalgesia.[9] If uncontrolled, the inflammatory process may result in exacerbation of the pain state following removal of the insult. Hence, the common goal with acute injury is to limit the inflammatory response, which in turn is likely to reduce discomfort.

Chronic Pain

Chronic pain is considered maladaptive when pain resulting from an acutely painful episode persists beyond the expected period of tissue healing. This maladaptive state progresses to cause alterations in physical components of the peripheral and central nervous systems, including changes to the membrane proteins, neurotransmitters, neuromodulators, and synaptic connectivity.[16] In horses this is recognized in musculoskeletal disease (eg, chronic laminitis, navicular disease); it is thought that pain perception is altered, resulting in increased sensitivity to noxious (hyperalgesia) and non-noxious (allodynia) stimuli.[9] Treatment of chronic pain states, therefore, generally requires a multifaceted approach.

TOOLS AVAILABLE TO ASSESS PAIN IN HORSES

Individualized subjective (eg, response to palpation) and semi-objective (eg, lameness grades, response to intra-articular medication) observational and interactive measures have been used by veterinarians to assess pain in horses. Issues surrounding these approaches include inconsistency between observers[17] and lack of universally applicable methods. Available tools and their limitations in obtaining repeatable and reliable results are described:

Physiologic Measurements

Heart rate, respiratory rate, temperature, blood pressure, beta-endorphins, and endogenous corticosteroids have all been measured in an effort to correlate with pain level.[6,18] These physiologic parameters, although easy to acquire and quantify, have been shown to have low sensitivity and specificity for pain in part because of multiple factors influencing these responses. For example, although pain may cause alterations in heart rate, other factors, such as shock, medications, stress, or exercise, may also be influential.[3,19] Physiologic parameters should, therefore, be assessed in conjunction with the remaining described measurements.

Observational and Interactive Methods

Behavior assessment

- Behavior assessment in the horse can be highly instructive if used carefully and applied systematically. This assessment may be used alone or as part of a composite scale.
- Behavior in the horse is influenced by temperament, age, sex, breed, and environment[20] necessitating individualized assessment. As interaction with people and other horses can alter demonstrated behavior, remote observation via closed circuit television (CCTV) or observation from a distance is recommended.
- Evaluations conducted in this manner should include demeanor, posture, and activity at rest. Signs of pain may include but are not limited to quietness, inappetence or reduced appetite, low head carriage, restlessness or frequent weight shifting, pointing a front limb or resting one limb, increased or reduced lying down, standing at the back of the stall, standing hunched over or stretched out, and looking at a painful area of the body.[18]
- Subtle signs that may be associated with pain, including bruxism, sweating, muscle fasciculations, and facial appearance, are observed in proximity to the horse.[21,22]
- Willingness to interact, and type of interaction, with a known owner/handler who is familiar with the horse's behaviors may provide additional information.
- Repeated behavioral assessment is often a useful marker during the initial investigation of a cause of musculoskeletal pain, for example, improvement in posture at rest or responsiveness during dynamic evaluation (eg, riding) following regional anesthesia and removal of pain.[23]

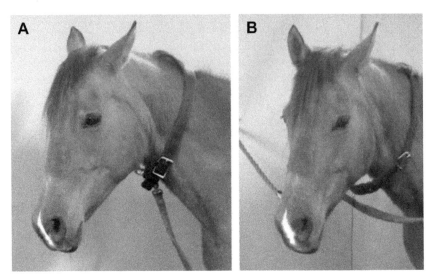

Fig. 1. (*A*) Horse during pain induction displaying low ears, an angled eye with an intense stare, mediolaterally dilated nostrils, and tension of the muzzle. (*B*) A horse during the control trial, relaxed with attentive ears and a relaxed stare. (*From* Gleerup KB, Forkman B, Lindegaard C, et al. An equine pain face. Vet Anaesth Analg 2014;42:111; with permission.)

Facial expression patterns

- Altered facial expression in response to varied stimuli has been recognized in the horse. Studies to document this and to determine if facial expressions in response to painful stimuli were consistent have been performed.[18,21,22]
- Observed via CCTV, the facial expressions most frequently associated with pain were low and/or asymmetrical ear positioning, an angled appearance of the eyes, a withdrawn or tense stare, mediolaterally dilated nostrils, and tension in the jaw, chin, lips, and certain facial muscles (**Fig. 1**).

Lameness grading

Lameness scales Veterinarians have used subjective lameness grading scales for many years. Several scales exist[24,25]; but often each veterinarian has their own criteria and their own application of the grading scale, based on personal clinical experience. The American Association of Equine Practitioners (AAEP) lameness grading scale is the most commonly used and is among the simplest and more repeatable (**Table 1**).

Lameness scale modifiers With the AAEP lameness grading scale veterinarians may assign a grade and additionally document the characteristics of the lameness to aid with repeatability of the observation; others have derived their own 0- to 8- or 0- to 10-point numerical scale.[26,27] Stride characteristics, such as abduction or adduction of the limb, toe drag, and weight shifting, can also be helpful.

Bilateral lameness may confound lameness assessment, as may the inability of the horse to trot because of significant lameness. Additionally, although scoring repeatability by the same examiner is high, interobserver repeatability is poor.[17] It has, therefore, been proposed that for improved validity the observer should be consistent between examinations and video recording of the examination with detailed

Table 1	
AAEP lameness scale	
Grade 0	Lameness not perceptible under any circumstances
Grade 1	Lameness is difficult to observe and is not consistently apparent, regardless of circumstances (eg, under saddle, circling, inclines, hard surfaces).
Grade 2	Lameness is difficult to observe at a walk or when trotting in a straight line but is consistently apparent under certain circumstances (eg, weight-carrying, circling, inclines, hard surfaces).
Grade 3	Lameness is consistently observable at a trot under all circumstances.
Grade 4	Lameness is obvious at a walk.
Grade 5	Lameness produces minimal weight bearing in motion and/or at rest or a complete inability to move.

From http://www.aaep.org/info/horse-health?publication=836. Accessed August 21, 2015. Copyright AEEP.

documentation of lameness characteristics should be included in medical records. Technology to objectively grade lameness (discussed later) is available.

Functional tests

Functional tests are incorporated in general clinical and dynamic examinations by most veterinarians (eg, flexion tests as part of lameness evaluation). The amount of flexion achieved, duration flexion is tolerated, and response to increased weight bearing on the stance limb provides useful information. Worsening lameness following flexion is assessed as increased or decreased and graded. Additional gait changes and contralateral limb response are also noted.

Pain scales

Results of studies detailing the development of composite pain scales for horses based on pain scoring systems used in humans and small animals are available.[28,29] Pain scales should be easy to use, broadly applicable and provide consistent and repeatable results.[28]

Composite pain scales frequently incorporate objective measurements (eg, physiologic parameters) with assessment of behavioral and interactive observations. An example of such a scale is one developed by Bussières and colleagues[28] for assessment of orthopedic pain following induction of tarsocrural joint osteoarthritis (**Table 2**). On re-evaluation by another research group,[29] consistency and interobserver repeatability were considered excellent under different study conditions.

Objective Methods

Biomechanical analysis

Kinetic and kinematic analysis are considered the gold standard approach to lameness evaluation and are increasingly used in research to document objective measurements of lameness with improved confidence.

Kinetics Kinetics is the study of forces acting on a body, for example, how forces generate motion in locomotion. Kinetic analysis is used in equine research to evaluate ground reaction force of each limb compared with another, with reduced ground reaction force correlating well with identified lameness. Typical patterns have been documented with respect to different types of lameness and replicated with high

Table 2
Multifactorial numerical rating composite pain scale for evaluating pain in horses

Physiologic Data	Criteria	Score: 12
Heart rate (compared with baseline)	<10% increase	0
	>11%–30% increase	1
	>31%–50% increase	2
	>50% increase	3
Respiratory rate (compared with baseline)	<10% increase	0
	>11%–30% increase	1
	>31%–50% increase	2
	>50% increase	3
Digestive sounds	Normal motility	0
	Decreased motility	1
	No motility	2
	Hypermotility	3
Rectal temperature (compared with baseline)	<0.5°C variation	0
	<1°C variation	1
	<2°C variation	2
	>2°C variation	3
Response to interaction	**Criteria**	**Score: 6**
Interactive behavior	Pays attention to people	0
	Exaggerated response to auditory stimuli	1
	Excessive to aggressive response to auditory stimuli	2
	Stupor, prostration, no response to auditory stimuli	3
Response to palpation of painful area	No reaction to palpation	0
	Mild reaction to palpation	1
	Resistance to palpation	2
	Violent reaction to palpation	3
Behavior	**Criteria**	**Score: 21**
Appearance (reluctance to move, restlessness, agitation, anxiety)	Bright, lowered head and ears, no reluctance to move	0
	Bright, alert, occasional head movement, no reluctance to move	1
	Restless, pricked up ears, abnormal facial expressions, dilated pupils	2
	Excited, continuous body movements, abnormal facial expression	3
Sweating	No obvious signs of sweat	0
	Damp to the touch	1
	Wet to the touch, beads of sweat apparent over body	2
	Excessive sweating, beads of sweat running off the animal	3
Kicking at abdomen	Quietly standing, no kicking	0
	Kicking at abdomen 1–2 times/5 min	1
	Kicking at abdomen 3–4 times/5 min	2
	Kicking at abdomen >5 times/5 min, intermittent attempts to roll	3
Pawing on floor (includes pointing or hanging limb)	Quietly standing, no pawing	0
	Occasionally pawing (1–2 times/5 min)	1
	Frequent pawing (3–4 times/5 min)	2
	Excessive pawing (>5 times/5 min)	3

(continued on next page)

Table 2 (continued)		
Posture (weight distribution and comfort)	Stands quietly, normal walk	0
	Occasional weight shift, slight muscle tremors	1
	Non–weight bearing, abnormal weight distribution	2
	Analgesic posture, attempts to urinate, prostration, muscle tremors	3
Head movement (lateral or vertical head movements)	No evidence of discomfort, head straight ahead mostly	0
	Intermittent head movement, looking at flanks or lip curl 1–2 times/5 min	1
	Intermittent, rapid head movement, looking at flanks or lip curl >5 times/5 min	2
	Continuous head movements, looking at flanks or lip curl >5 times/5 min	3
Appetite	Eats hay readily	0
	Hesitates to eat hay	1
	Little interest in eating hay, takes hay but does not chew or swallow	2
	Neither shows interest in nor eats hay	3
Total CPS		39

From Bussières G, Jacques C, Lainay O, et al. Development of a composite orthopaedic pain scale in horses. Res Vet Sci 2008;85(2):296–7; with permission from Elsevier.

repeatability.[30] Limitations to this method of gait analysis do exist and should be considered with respect to the clinical or research scenario. Several methods of kinetic data collection have been developed: the static force plate, the dynamometric horseshoe, in-shoe measurement systems,[31,32] and the hoof wall strain gauge.[33] The most valuable resource for measuring equine kinetic data currently is the force measuring equine treadmill at the University of Zurich,[34] a custom-built facility that has provided invaluable information on this subject.

Kinematics Kinematics is the study of movement of a body. This information is used to generate information on motion characteristics of the limb through the stride phases to establish range and duration of motion of each joint within the limb. Changes have been reported to correlate well with specific alterations in gait.[8] Kinematics are more easily measured than kinetics, and equipment is less expensive allowing for its broader use in clinical settings.

Gait analysis technology Clinical applications of kinematic technology have been developed for lameness examinations using inertial sensors alongside an accelerometer to document movement symmetry.[8] Commercial systems suggest suitability for use at the trot in a straight line, in a circle, and after blocking; programs established for different surface types are also part of the standard package.

Goniometery
Goniometery may be used to assess joint range of motion through a rehabilitation program and may be particularly useful in horses with advanced joint disease or those with lordosis of the thoracolumbar spine.[35]

Pressure algometry
Pressure algometry has been shown to provide reliable and repeated objective assessment of mechanical nociception thresholds in studies investigating thoracic

limb pain associated with induced synovitis or osteoarthritis, muscle pain, mechanical nociceptive thresholds of the pastern region and the axial skeleton, and to measure the effect of sedative drugs in the provision of analgesia[7,36] This technique is used increasingly in research studies investigating pain and has been suggested for use in the objective clinical evaluation of axial skeleton pain.[4,37] Pressure-calibrated hoof testers have been used to quantify pain in laminitic horses.

Thermography
Thermography documents skin and superficial tissue temperature, providing reference for identification and monitoring of sites of inflamed or injured tissue. Limitations include environmental influence (eg, sensitivity to drafts, sunlight).[38]

Response to Treatment

Diagnostic anesthesia
Intra-articular or regional anesthesia and subsequent assessment may be performed to localize the source of pain before diagnostic imaging and treatment. Although multiple limb lameness can confound results, this tool is still of value and use may be enhanced by dynamic evaluation (eg, under saddle).

Response to medication
Although a less direct evaluation of pain, this method is used for horses when circumstances limit a thorough work-up and may include systemic or regional medications. In addition to the potential for inappropriate treatment, there is a potential to worsen the pathological condition.

MODULATION OF PAIN IN EQUINE PATIENTS

Research evaluating the efficacy of analgesia provided by different therapeutic modalities in the horse is limited. Often articles of studies show a lack of appropriate inclusion of control groups, and several demonstrate investigator bias. Others involve only research horses with induced pain at focal sites, limiting the capacity to draw conclusions on the effect of analgesics in clinically painful conditions and more so with chronic pain states. To ensure the best outcome, treatment of pain should be based on the likely mechanism of action causing pain and aim specifically at targeted improvement (eg, anti-inflammatory, nerve regeneration) and then further tailored according to response.[39] The next section focuses on how treatment modalities provide pain modulation in equine patients with musculoskeletal pain. The interested reader is referred to additional sources for more detail.[40–42]

Pharmacologic Options

Nonsteroidal anti-inflammatory drugs
Nonsteroidal anti-inflammatory drugs (NSAIDs) are commonly used via intravenous (IV) or oral routes. Phenylbutazone, flunixin meglumine, firocoxib, ketoprofen, aspirin, and diclofenac are licensed for use in the United States. NSAIDs inhibit cyclooxygenase to reduce concentration of prostaglandins PGE_2, PGI_2, and thromboxane A_2 (TXA_2) within tissues, providing a local anti-inflammatory effect and dampening down peripheral sensitization. Excellent analgesic efficacy, alone or in combination with other pharmacologic agents, is reported.[43,44] There is no current evidence for combining NSAIDs in the management of pain in horses.[45] Adverse effects include gastrointestinal tract ulceration (particularly in foals), nephrotoxicity, and hepatotoxicity.

Corticosteroids

Triamcinolone and methylprednisolone are among medications administered intra-articularly for anti-inflammatory effects mediated by inhibition of phospholipase A_2. Although efficacious when used correctly, adverse effects include systemically reduced glycosaminoglycan concentrations in joints,[46] immunosuppression, and laminitis.[47]

Opioids

Although many drugs with actions at mu and/or kappa receptors are available, use of systemic opioids for analgesia in horses remains controversial as clear benefits have not been elucidated and side effects (eg, gastrointestinal stasis, excitation) with escalation in dose are of concern. When administered via alternative routes (eg, epidural, intra-articular), efficacy is demonstrated[48,49] and adverse effects are fewer. These considerations and the need for strict record keeping will likely limit opioid use to the hospital setting where monitoring is more frequent and additional drugs may be used in conjunction.

Tramadol

Currently investigations of pharmacodynamics and pharmacokinetics of this codeine analogue following oral and IV administration do not support its use as an analgesic in horses.

Alpha-2 agonists

Alpha-2 agonists decrease neuronal excitation by activating presynaptic and postsynaptic alpha-2 receptors in the descending inhibitory pain pathway centrally and in joints peripherally.[41] Clinically used most commonly for sedation, alpha-2 adrenoceptor agonists are also good analgesics and in acute conditions supplement a multimodal approach to analgesia. Sole or chronic use is limited by sedative, musculoskeletal (eg, ataxia), and physiologic effects (eg, bradycardia, sweating, respiratory gastrointestinal stasis).

Local anesthetics

This class of drugs may be administered regionally (eg, intra-articular, perineural) or systemically (lidocaine) for pain management. When regionally administered, local anesthetic drugs block sodium channels, thereby preventing conduction through sensory nerve fibers. Efficacy may be affected by low tissue pH as with inflammation[50]; although adverse effects are limited, detrimental effects on articular cartilage are reported and warrant further investigation.[51] When systemically administered, data support lidocaine's anti-inflammatory and analgesic effects[50]; however, because of its short action it must be given by IV infusion. If dosed inappropriately, systemic administration of lidocaine can result in hypotension, seizures, and collapse; bupivacaine is not recommended for systemic IV use because of reported cardiovascular toxicity.

Ketamine

Noncompetitive N-methyl-D-aspartate (NMDA) antagonism by ketamine limits binding of the excitatory neurotransmitter glutamate to NMDA channels, inhibiting potentiation of action potentials within the sensory central nervous system. Via this mechanism ketamine is thought to reduce the occurrence of wind up (increased responsiveness), hyperalgesia, and central sensitization that results from chronic or continuous noxious stimulation of polymodal C nociceptive afferent nerve fibers.[40] Ketamine is used extensively as a general anesthetic and in limited circumstances as an adjunct to alpha-2/opioid sedation for standing procedures. The elimination half-life of ketamine is approximately 1 hour,[52] again necessitating its administration via constant rate infusion, although other routes are described (eg, epidural, intramuscular). Adverse effects include hyperexcitability, muscle tremors, tachycardia, tachypnea, and ataxia.[53]

Gabapentin
Gabapentin is an anticonvulsant drug that has shown promise in human and small animal patients as a treatment of neuropathic pain. Gabapentin is rapidly absorbed and has an elimination half-life of 3.4 hours in horses. Although the collective experience with this drug in horses is limited, reports indicate there may be possible benefits.

Polysulfated glycosaminoglycans
Polysulfated glycosaminoglycans (PSGAGs) are used in clinical practice for the treatment of joint-associated pain via intramuscular administration or intra-articular injection. PSGAGs have been reported to decrease inflammatory mediators, including PGE2 and upregulate collagen synthesis in joints.[54] In a study on the effects of PSGAGs on induced osteoarthritis of the carpus, lameness grading improved with treatment and joint effusion decreased compared with controls, suggesting anti-inflammatory properties.

Sarapin
A distillate of powdered *Sarracenia purpurea* (pitcher plant), Sarapin has been advocated as an analgesic in chronic pain, especially if of neural origin despite the method of action being unknown.[39] In equine patients, Sarapin is used for the treatment of muscle pain associated with the thoracolumbar spine and for infiltration around the sacroiliac joints. No known side effects have been documented following such use.

Interventional Therapies

Interventional therapies have become increasingly available in recent years, with advances in sports medicine research in the human and equine field. The following therapeutic options have been covered elsewhere in this text and so are discussed only with respect to provision of analgesia.

Manual therapy
This therapy focuses on alleviating sensory, neuromuscular, and mechanical abnormalities. Pain is modulated along with proprioceptive and motor retraining. Therapeutic exercises are designed to be specific to the function of the injured tissue[35] and aimed at reparative or healing processes within the neuromusculoskeletal system.[55] Examples of different modalities within this broad group are listed:

Chiropractic Chiropractic treatment is characterized by high-velocity, low-amplitude thrusts, applied to the spine[56] and has been shown to reduce spinal pain.[4] Chiropractic induced a 27% increase in mechanical nociceptive thresholds for up to 7 days compared with baseline in a clinical trial comparing changes in mechanical nociceptive thresholds in response to pharmacologic and nonpharmacologic therapies.[57] The specific mechanisms of analgesia are not well known; however, influences on biomechanical, physiologic, neurologic, and psychological mechanisms[58] have been proposed. Long-term benefits are thought to occur via actions on the ascending and descending pain-modulating spinal cord pathways.[59]

Physiotherapy Physiotherapy refers to passive or assisted active movements applied to address impairments in the articular, neural, and muscular systems.[60] Ongoing research into the analgesic mechanism underlying physiotherapy suggests that focally induced movement may activate afferent neurons and stimulate neural inhibitory systems at multiple spinal levels, producing hypoalgesia.[61] Passive accessory mobilization of the cervical spine (as compared with placebo) has been demonstrated to provide pain relief in specific conditions.[62] Similar benefits of physiotherapy are reported in people.[63]

Massage Although there are limited case-controlled data to support clinical observations of improvement in pain states following massage, studies have demonstrated an increased mechanical nociceptive threshold in the thoracolumbar region[57] and improved stride lengths at walk and trot[64] after massage. Tissue manipulation effects changes in neurologic signaling relating to pain processing and motor control[60] and upregulates signaling within large-diameter nerve fibers to provide inhibition of the ascending nociceptive signals.[65] Soft tissue mobilization improves blood flow improving tissue viability and so reduces pain associated with tissue damage.[66] Release of endorphins and serotonin via these mechanisms may also modulate pain perception.

Therapeutic exercise Exercises, such as hand walking, walking over poles, backing, and hill work, aim to return the soft tissues and bones to normal physical capacity. Sensory, neuromotor, and mechanical abnormalities that occur as a consequence of injury may be alleviated by the analgesic effects of therapeutic exercise.[35] However, alternative pain modulation may also be necessary to ensure that therapeutic exercises are executed optimally.

Other Therapeutic Modalities

Hydrotherapy
In people, aquatic therapies have been reported to decrease pain[67]; it is shown that exercising in water has beneficial effects through the following mechanisms[68]:

Buoyancy Buoyancy reduces weight bearing of the affected limb and, thus, secondary compensation; it also allows increased joint stability.[69]

Hydrostatic pressure Circumferential compression is achieved by immersion in water, and the effects are proportional to water depth. Increases in hydrostatic pressure allow increased circulation and reduction of tissue edema.[67]

Tissue temperature Increasing water temperature provides stimulus for increased circulation and decreased muscle spasm in warm water[70] and in cold-water stimulus for vasoconstriction to reduce the influx of inflammatory mediators.[71]

Hydrotherapy, therefore, provides significant opportunity for analgesia in the rehabilitation period through reduction of local tissue edema and inflammation to reduce pressure, thermal and chemical nociceptive stimulation, and via periods of off-weighting the injured tissues, in static and dynamic conditions, such that therapeutic exercise can be achieved in minimally loaded conditions.

Cryotherapy
Ice packs, ice boots, ice-water circulating boots, cold hosing, and products, such as the Game Ready (Game Ready, Concord, California), can deliver cold therapy, making cryotherapy very accessible. Cold therapy is most beneficial when applied immediately after injury and reapplied every 2 to 4 hours. Cold therapy provides analgesia to an area of injury by initiation of local vasoconstriction, decreasing vascular permeability, reducing the influx of inflammatory markers to the area, depressing neuronal conductivity, and decreasing the metabolic rate, thereby reducing cell hypoxia and death.[72] Cryotherapy has been demonstrated to reduce the activity of enzymatic mediators of acute laminitis in the horse.[73]

Acupuncture

Acupuncture is effective for treating pain[74] via release of locally active neuropeptides, which initiate a systemic analgesic response mediated by endogenous opioid peptides, serotonin, dopamine, and norepinephrine after needle placement or acupressure.[75] Increased concentrations of endogenous opioids in plasma and cerebrospinal fluid following acupuncture have been documented in the horse.[76]

Electroacupuncture has been demonstrated in humans to significantly increase mechanical and thermal pain thresholds over manual and sham acupuncture in healthy patients.[77] In horses, a series of 3 electroacupuncture treatments has been shown to resolve chronic thoracolumbar spine pain.[78] The mechanism of analgesia for chronic pain states with electroacupuncture seems to be mediated via endogenous opioid peptides, β-endorphin and cortisol.[76]

Low-level laser therapy

Protocols for treatment of wounds, tendinitis, desmitis, osteoarthritis and muscular soreness are available for horses. A systematic review of studies evaluating low level laser therapy in human osteoarthritis suggests a positive analgesic effect when the recommended low level laser therapy guidelines were adhered to.[79] It is postulated that analgesia for osteoarthritis is the result of inhibiting inflammation of the joint capsule and is therefore reliant on appropriate patient and energy selection.[80]

Extracorporeal shockwave therapy

Extracorporeal shockwave therapy has been shown to have modifying effects in induced carpal osteoarthritis models.[81] Initial analgesic effects were demonstrated to last 2 to 3 days, but overall improvements in lameness score and range of motion were observed 14 days after treatment. In humans extracorporeal shockwave therapy has been successful at reducing pain and improving healing in chronic plantar fasciitis[82] and chronic low back pain.[83] The origin of the analgesic effect is unclear,[84] but it is thought that extracorporeal shockwave therapy induces neovascularization and reactivation of healing in damaged tendons, ligaments and bone.[85] Analgesia may also be provided by appropriate motor stimulation of muscles and tendons through application of extracorporeal shockwave therapy.[83]

Transcutaneous electrical nerve stimulation

Electrotherapy provides pain relief through transduction of electrical current into the body to depolarize sensory neurons to suppress pain.[86] Analgesic efficacy is variable, but TENS has been demonstrated to provide excellent short-term relief from chronic pain in humans. TENS is used with similar perceived effects in the horse, but to date no scientific basis for treatment has been documented.

Therapeutic ultrasound

Ultrasound waves produce thermal and nonthermal effects on tissues to improve local circulation, increase cell membrane permeability, enhance collagen extensibility and reduce muscle spasm.[86,87] Increased pain thresholds are hypothesized to be due to vasodilation, increasing intracellular calcium and/or increasing fibrous tissue extensibility.[86,88] Use in the horse is increasing in popularity, with treatment effects inferred from studies in human and small animals.

Kinesiotaping

Despite a recent review concluding that there is no substantial evidence for analgesic efficacy of kinesiotaping in humans[89] it is still extensively used in people and increasingly in horses. Taping provides release of pressure on tissues from skin and increases space for movement of lymphatic fluid.[89] It is proposed that the application of kinesiotape provides consistent mechanical stimulation to downregulate nociceptive transmission.[90] Its usefulness in horses is undocumented.

SUMMARY

Although there is much to do to improve our evaluation and management of equine pain, advances are ongoing and newer modalities for diagnosis and therapy are increasingly available.

REFERENCES

1. Merskey H, Bogduk N. Part III: pain terms, a current list with definitions and notes on usage. In: Merskey H, Bogduk N, editors. Classification of chronic pain, descriptors of chronic pain syndromes and definitions of pain terms. 2nd edition. Seattle (WA): IASP Press; 1994.
2. Ashley FH, Waterman-Pearson AE, Whay HR. Behavioural assessment of pain in horses and donkeys: application to clinical practice and future studies. Equine Vet J 2005;37(6):565–75.
3. Taylor PM, Pascoe PJ, Mama KR. Diagnosing and treating pain in the horse. Where are we today? Vet Clin North Am Equine Pract 2002;18(1):1–19.
4. Haussler KK, Erb HN. Pressure algometry: objective assessment of back pain and effects of chiropractic treatment. 49th Annu Conv Am Assoc Equine Pract 2003;49:2–6.
5. Wennerstrand J, Johnston C, Roethlisberger-Holm K, et al. Kinematic evaluation of the back in the sport horse with back pain. Equine Vet J 2004;36(8): 707–11.
6. Raekallio M, Taylor PM, Bennett RC. Preliminary investigations of pain and analgesia assessment in horses administered phenylbutazone or placebo after arthroscopic surgery. Vet Surg 1997;26(2):150–5.
7. Love EJ, Murrell J, Whay HR. Thermal and mechanical nociceptive threshold testing in horses: a review. Vet Anaesth Analg 2011;38(1):3–14.
8. Keegan KG. Evidence-based lameness detection and quantification. Vet Clin North Am Equine Pract 2007;23(2):403–23.
9. Sandkühler J. Models and mechanisms of hyperalgesia and allodynia. Physiol Rev 2009;89(2):707–58.
10. Meyer RA, Ringkamp M, Campbell JN, et al. Peripheral mechanisms of cutaneous nociception. In: McMahon SB, Koltzenburg M, editors. Wall and Melzack's textbook of pain 5th edition, vol 1, 5th edition. London: Elsevier Ltd; 2006. p. 3–34.
11. Todd AJ, Koerber HR. Neuroanatomical substrates of spinal nociception. In: McMahon SB, Koltzenburg M, editors. Wall and Melzack's textbook of pain 5th edition, vol 1, 5th edition. London: Elsevier Ltd; 2006. p. 73–90.
12. Melzack R, Wall PD. Pain mechanisms: a new theory. Science 1965;150:971–9.
13. Chudler EH, Anton F, Dubner R, et al. Responses of nociceptive SI neurons in monkeys and pain sensation in humans elicited by noxious thermal stimulation. J Neurophysiol 1990;63:559–69.
14. Saab CY, Willis WD. The cerebellum: Organization, functions and its role in nociception. Brain Res Rev 2003;42(1):85–95.
15. Fields HL, Basbaum AI, Heinricher MM. Central nervous system mechanisms of pain modulation. In: McMahon SB, Koltzenburg M, editors. Wall and Melzack's textbook of pain, vol 1, 5th edition. London: Elsevier Ltd; 2003. p. 125–42.

16. Fairbanks CA, Goracke-Postle CJ. Neurobiological studies of chronic pain and analgesia: rationale and refinements. Eur J Pharmacol 2015;759:169–81.

17. Fuller CJ, Bladon BM, Driver AJ, et al. The intra- and inter-assessor reliability of measurement of functional outcome by lameness scoring in horses. Vet J 2006; 171(2):281–6.

18. Love E. Equine Pain Management. In: Auer JA, Stick JA, editors. Equine Surgery, vol 1, 4th Edition. St. Louis: Elsevier Saunders; 2012. p. 263–70.

19. Wagner AE. Effects of stress on pain in horses and incorporating pain scales for equine practice. Vet Clin North Am Equine Pract 2010;26(3):481–92.

20. De Grauw JC, van Loon JPAM. Systematic pain assessment in horses. Vet J 2015. http://dx.doi.org/10.1016/j.tvjl.2015.07.030.

21. Gleerup KB, Forkman B, Lindegaard C, et al. An equine pain face. Vet Anaesth Analg 2014;42(1):103–14.

22. Dalla Costa E, Minero M, Lebelt D, et al. Development of the Horse Grimace Scale (HGS) as a pain assessment tool in horses undergoing routine castration. PLoS One 2014;9(3):e92281.

23. Barstow A, Dyson S. Clinical features and diagnosis of sacroiliac joint region pain in 296 horses: 2004-2014. Equine Vet Educ 2015;1–11. http://dx.doi.org/10.1111/eve.12377.

24. Wyn-Jones G. Equine lameness. In: Wyn-Jones G, editor. Equine Lameness. 1st edition. Oxford (United Kingdom): Blackwell Scientific; 1988.

25. American association of equine practitioners. AAEP guidelines for lameness evaluation. 2015. Available at: http://www.aaep.org/info/horse-health?publication=836. Accessed August 21, 2015.

26. Dyson S. Recognition of lameness: man versus machine. Vet J 2014;201(3):245–8.

27. Ramzan PHL, Palmer L, Powell SE. Unicortical condylar fracture of the Thoroughbred fetlock: 45 cases (2006-2013). Equine Vet J 2014;10:1–4.

28. Bussières G, Jacques C, Lainay O, et al. Development of a composite orthopaedic pain scale in horses. Res Vet Sci 2008;85(2):294–306.

29. Van Loon JPAM, Back W, Hellebrekers LJ, et al. Application of a composite pain scale to objectively monitor horses with somatic and visceral pain under hospital conditions. J Equine Vet Sci 2010;30(11):641–9.

30. Weishaupt MA. Adaptation strategies of horses with lameness. Vet Clin North Am Equine Pract 2008;24(1):79–100.

31. Judy CE, Galuppo LD, Snyder JR, et al. Evaluation of an in-shoe pressure measurement system in horses. Am J Vet Res 2001;62(1):23–8.

32. Chateau H, Robin D, Simonelli T, et al. Design and validation of a dynamometric horseshoe for the measurement of three-dimensional ground reaction force on a moving horse. J Biomech 2009;42(3):336–40.

33. Thomason JJ, Peterson ML. Biomechanical and mechanical investigations of the hoof-track interface in racing horses. Vet Clin North Am Equine Pract 2008;24(1):53–77.

34. Weishaupt MA, Hogg HP, Wiestner T, et al. Instrumented treadmill for measuring vertical ground reaction forces in horses. Am J Vet Res 2002;63(4):520–7.

35. Paulekas R, Haussler KK. Principles and practice of therapeutic exercise for horses. J Equine Vet Sci 2009;29(12):870–93.

36. Taylor PM, Crosignani N, Lopes C, et al. Mechanical nociceptive thresholds using four probe configurations in horses. Vet Anaesth Analg 2015;1–10. http://dx.doi.org/10.1111/vaa.12274.

37. Haussler KK. Functional assessment and rehabilitation of the equine axial skeleton. Am Coll Vet Surg Symp 2012;1:175–84.

38. Tunley BV, Henson FMD. Reliability and repeatability of thermographic examination and the normal thermographic image of the thoracolumbar region in the horse. Equine Vet J 2004;36(4):306–12.
39. Muir WW. Pain: mechanisms and management in horses. Vet Clin North Am Equine Pract 2010;26(3):467–80.
40. Muir WW. NMDA receptor antagonists and pain: ketamine. Vet Clin North Am Equine Pract 2010;26(3):565–78.
41. Valverde A. Alpha-2 agonists as pain therapy in horses. Vet Clin North Am Equine Pract 2010;26(3):515–32.
42. Clutton RE. Opioid analgesia in horses. Vet Clin North Am Equine Pract 2010; 26(3):493–514.
43. Foreman JH, Grubb TL, Inoue OJ, et al. Efficacy of single-dose intravenous phenylbutazone and flunixin meglumine before, during and after exercise in an experimental reversible model of foot lameness in horses. Equine Vet J 2010; 42(Suppl 38):601–5.
44. Thomasy SM, Slovis N, Maxwell LK, et al. Transdermal fentanyl combined with nonsteroidal anti-inflammatory drugs for analgesia in horses. J Vet Intern Med 2004;18(4):550–4.
45. Keegan KG, Messer NT, Reed SK, et al. Effectiveness of administration of phenylbutazone alone or concurrent administration of phenylbutazone and flunixin meglumine to alleviate lameness in horses. Am J Vet Res 2008;69(2): 167–73.
46. Frisbie DD, Kawcak CE, Baxter GM, et al. Effects of 6-alpha-methylprednisolone acetate on an equine osteochondral fragment exercise model. Am J Vet Res 1998;59(12):1619–28.
47. Bailey SR, Elliott J. The corticosteroid laminitis story: 2. Science of if, when and how. Equine Vet J 2007;39(1):7–11.
48. Lindegaard C, Thomsen MH, Larsen S, et al. Analgesic efficacy of intra-articular morphine in experimentally induced radiocarpal synovitis in horses. Vet Anaesth Analg 2010;37(2):171–85.
49. Goodrich LR, Nixon AJ, Fubini SL, et al. Epidural morphine and detomidine decreases postoperative hindlimb lameness in horses after bilateral stifle arthroscopy. Vet Surg 2002;31(3):232–9.
50. Doherty TJ, Seddighi MR. Local anesthetics as pain therapy in horses. Vet Clin North Am Equine Pract 2010;26(3):533–49.
51. Piat P, Richard H, Beauchamp G, et al. In vivo effects of a single intra-articular injection of 2% lidocaine or 0.5% bupivacaine on articular cartilage of normal horses. Vet Surg 2012;41(8):1002–10.
52. Kaka JS, Klavano PA, Hayton WL. Pharmacokinetics of ketamine in the horse. Am J Vet Res 1979;40(7):978–81.
53. Wagner AE, Mama KR, Contino EK, et al. Evaluation of sedation and analgesia in standing horses after administration of xylazine, butorphanol, and subanesthetic doses of ketamine. J Am Vet Med Assoc 2011;238:1629–33.
54. Frisbie DD, McIlwraith CW, Kawcak CE, et al. Evaluation of intra-articular hyaluronan, sodium chondroitin sulfate and N-acetyl-d-glucosamine combination versus saline (0.9% NaCl) for osteoarthritis using an equine model. Vet J 2013; 197(3):824–9.
55. Haussler KK. The role of manual therapies in equine pain management. Vet Clin North Am Equine Pract 2010;26(3):579–601.
56. Maigne JY, Vautravers P. Mechanism of action of spinal manipulative therapy. Joint Bone Spine 2003;70(5):336–41.

57. Sullivan KA, Hill AE, Haussler KK. The effects of chiropractic, massage and phenylbutazone on spinal mechanical nociceptive thresholds in horses without clinical signs. Equine Vet J 2008;40(1):14–20.

58. Pickar JG. Neurophysiological effects of spinal manipulation. Spine J 2002;2(5): 357–71.

59. Boal RW, Gillette RG. Central neuronal plasticity, low back pain and spinal manipulative therapy. J Manipulative Physiol Ther 2004;27(5):314–26.

60. Goff LM. Manual therapy for the horse-a contemporary perspective. J Equine Vet Sci 2009;29(11):799–808.

61. Wright A. Hypoalgesia post-manipulative therapy: a review of a potential neurophysiological mechanism. Man Ther 1995;1:11–6.

62. Vicenzino B, Collins D, Benson H, et al. An investigation of the interrelationship between manipulative therapy-induced hypoalgesia and sympathoexcitation. J Manipulative Physiol Ther 1998;21(7):448–53.

63. Moss P, Sluka K, Wright A. The initial effects of knee joint mobilization on osteoarthritic hyperalgesia. Man Ther 2007;12(2):109–18.

64. Wilson J. The effects of sports massage on athletic performance and general function. Massage Ther J 2002;41(2):90–101.

65. Imamura M, Furlan AD, Dryden T, et al. Evidence-informed management of chronic low back pain with massage. Spine J 2008;8(1):121–33.

66. Weerapong P, Hume PA, Kolt GS. The mechanisms of massage and effects on performance, muscle recovery and injury prevention. Sports Med 2005;35(3): 235–56.

67. Kamioka H, Tsutani K, Mutoh Y, et al. A systematic review of nonrandomized controlled trials on the curative effects of aquatic exercise. Int J Gen Med 2011;4:239–60.

68. King MR, Haussler KK, Kawcak CE, et al. Mechanisms of aquatic therapy and its potential use in managing equine osteoarthritis. Equine Vet Educ 2013;25(4): 204–9.

69. Hinman RS, Heywood SE, Day AR. Aquatic physical therapy for hip and knee osteoarthritis: results of a single-blind randomized controlled trial. Phys Ther 2007;87(1):32–43.

70. Yamazaki F, Endo Y, Torii R, et al. Continuous monitoring of change in hemodilution during water immersion in humans: effect of water temperature. Aviat Space Environ Med 2000;71(6):632–9.

71. Buchner HHF, Schildboeck U. Physiotherapy applied to the horse: a review. Equine Vet J 2006;38(6):574–80.

72. Michlovitz SL. Thermal agents in rehabilitation. In: Michlovitz SL, editor. 3rd edition. Philadelphia, PA: FA Davis; 1996.

73. Worster AA, Gaughan EM, Hoskinson JJ, et al. Effects of external thermal manipulation on laminar temperature and perfusion scintigraphy of the equine digit. N Z Vet J 2000;48(4):111–6.

74. Fry LM, Neary S, Sharrock J, et al. Acupuncture for analgesia in veterinary medicine. Top Companion Anim Med 2014;29(2):35–42.

75. Yoo YC, Oh JH, Kwon TD, et al. Analgesic mechanism of electroacupuncture in an arthritic pain model of rats: a neurotransmitter study. Yonsei Med J 2011; 52(6):1016–21.

76. Skarda RT, Tejwani GA, Muir WW 3rd. Cutaneous analgesia, hemodynamic and respiratory effects, and beta-endorphin concentration in spinal fluid and plasma of horses after acupuncture and electroacupuncture. Am J Vet Res 2002;63(10): 1435–42.

77. Baeumler PI, Fleckenstein J, Takayama S, et al. Effects of acupuncture on sensory perception: A systematic review and meta-analysis. Deutsche Zeitschrift fur Akupunktur 58, 29;2015.
78. Xie H, Colahan P, Ott EA. Evaluation of electroacupuncture treatment of horses with signs of chronic thoracolumbar pain. J Am Vet Med Assoc 2005;227(2): 281–6.
79. Jang H, Lee H. Meta-analysis of pain relief effects by laser irradiation on joint areas. Photomed Laser Surg 2012;30(8):405–17.
80. Bjordal JM, Couppé C, Chow RT, et al. A systematic review of low level laser therapy with location-specific doses for pain from chronic joint disorders: Aust J Physiother 2003;49(2):107–16.
81. Frisbie DD, Kawcak CE, McIlwraith CW. Evaluation of the effect of extracorporeal shock wave treatment on experimentally induced osteoarthritis in middle carpal joints of horses. Am J Vet Res 2009;70(4):449–54.
82. Vahdatpour B, Sajadieh S, Bateni V, et al. Extracorporeal shock wave therapy in patients with plantar fasciitis. A randomized, placebo-controlled trial with ultrasonographic and subjective outcome assessments. J Res Med Sci 2012;17(9): 834–8.
83. Han H, Lee D, Lee S, et al. The effects of extracorporeal shock wave therapy on pain, disability, and depression of chronic low back pain patients. J Phys Ther Sci 2015;27:397–9.
84. McCure SR, Dahlberg JA, Abed JM, et al. Continuing study of analgesia resulting from extracorporeal shock wave therapy. Analgesia 2006;52:583–4.
85. Wang C-J. Extracorporeal shockwave therapy in musculoskeletal disorders. J Orthop Surg Res 2012;7(1):11.
86. Steiss JE, Levine D. Physical agent modalities. Vet Clin North Am Small Anim Pract 2005;35(6):1317–33.
87. Baker KG, Robertson VJ, Duck FA. A review of therapeutic ultrasound: biophysical effects. Phys Ther 2001;81(7):1351–8.
88. Ozgönenel L, Aytekin E, Durmuşoglu G. A double-blind trial of clinical effects of therapeutic ultrasound in knee osteoarthritis. Ultrasound Med Biol 2009;35(1): 44–9.
89. Morris D, Jones D, Ryan H, et al. The clinical effects of Kinesio Tex taping: a systematic review. Physiother Theory Pract 2013;29(4):259–70.
90. Bassett KT, Lingman SA, Ellis RF. The use and treatment efficacy of kinaesthetic taping for musculoskeletal conditions: a systematic review. NZ J Physiother 2010; 38(2):56–62.

Physiotherapy Assessment for the Equine Athlete

Lesley Goff, PhD, MAnimSt(AnimPhysio), MAppSc(ExSpSc), GDipManip, BAppSc(Physio)[a,b,c,*]

KEYWORDS

- Equine physiotherapy • Assessment • Functional • Palpation

KEY POINTS

- Equine physiotherapists take a functional approach to the assessment of the horse, using clinical reasoning through all stages of the assessment.
- Equine physiotherapists are consulted when there is a movement dysfunction or poor performance, which may or may not be directly associated with the diagnosed condition.
- Equine physiotherapists try to use an evidence-based approach to their assessment, which includes the use of outcome measures.

INTRODUCTION

Physiotherapy assessment of the equine athlete involves an extrapolation to the horse, of the skills that these practitioners have developed in their training and practice as human physiotherapists. Unlike veterinarians, physiotherapists do not require a pathoanatomic diagnosis to develop a treatment plan.[1] In contrast, physiotherapists use a more functional approach to assessment of the horse by way of observing and identifying movement dysfunctions or impairments, and using their clinical reasoning to relate what they observe and also palpate to the presenting problem. This article gives the reader some insight into the subjective physiotherapy assessment and the physiotherapist's physical examination of the equine athlete. Outcome measures are also discussed. It is beyond the scope of this article to include a discussion of the equine physiotherapist's important role in assessing the horse–rider unit.

The author has nothing to disclose.

[a] Active Animal Physiotherapy, P.O. Box 277, Highfields, Queensland 4352, Australia; [b] Equine Science, School of Agriculture and Food Sciences, Faculty of Science, University of Queensland, Gatton, 4345, Queensland, Australia; [c] Faculty of Health and Life Sciences, School of Veterinary Science, University of Liverpool, Liverpool, UK

* Active Animal Physiotherapy, P.O. Box 277, Highfields, Queensland 4352, Australia.

E-mail address: lesley@animalphysio.com.au

The Basis of Equine Physiotherapy Assessment

It is paramount, when devising and delivering any form of treatment or management of the equine athlete, to have a comprehensive assessment process. Skills that are useful for a comprehensive physiotherapy assessment are listed below:

- Good communication with the owner, handler, and trainer;
- Good powers of observation (static and dynamic);
- Knowledge of anatomy, functional anatomy, and biomechanics of the horse;
- The ability to perform or direct functional movement tests;
- Good palpation skills; and
- The ability to interpret all of these assessments.

The process of interpreting all these parameters is clinical reasoning, or problem solving, and is an essential part of the each step of the equine athlete assessment.[1] Communication is one of the critical skills required to develop good clinical reasoning,[2] and has been linked with significant outcomes of care, including accuracy, efficiency, supportiveness, adherence to treatment plans, and client and veterinarian satisfaction.[2] Communication includes determining the problem that the owner, handler, or trainer perceives as existing in their equine athlete, and what they wish to have assessed and managed. The owner, handler, or trainer should have a preliminary veterinary diagnosis for any conditions or diseases that exist in the horse.

Often, physiotherapists are consulted when there is a movement dysfunction or poor performance, which may or may not be associated directly with the condition that has been diagnosed. An example of such a situation is that of a horse with healed fracture of the orbital socket, which had been caused by a traumatic accident involving the horse pulling back and striking the area of the head on a metal pole. The diagnosis was the fracture, and reconstructive surgery was performed. Three months later, the fracture was healed and horse seemed to have recovered well, yet the horse demonstrated an inability to flex laterally in either direction on a small circle, owing to segmental hypomobility in the midcervical spine. The latter may have occurred during the traumatic incident, yet was not part of the original diagnosis.

Therefore, after the diagnosis is given by the veterinarian, it is important for the physiotherapist to take an extensive clinical history to document the degree of functional disability perceived, onset and progression of the disorder, and the past history related to the disorder.[1] Taking a history requires good interpersonal skills as well as a good knowledge base. Time spent with the owner obtaining information allows the physiotherapist to observe the animal's general demeanor and behavior while observing its general condition, conformation, gait, and posture.[1]

When performing a physiotherapy assessment for the equine athlete, the structure of a history may include the following (adapted from Goff[1]):

- Recording of the area affected/effect of dysfunction;
- Current veterinary diagnosis;
- Current perceived impairment or movement dysfunction;
- Past history (including past treatments);
- Questions to determine contraindications and precautions to treatment;
- Questions related to the equine athlete's sport (including equipment and tack used);
- Owner and handler expectations of future occupation or activity; and
- For ridden horses, questions related to rider biomechanics and existing injuries.

OBSERVATION

Along with communication, clinical reasoning begins with the physiotherapist's interpretation of clues from the patient. These initial clues help the physiotherapist to formulate a preliminary working hypothesis. The working hypothesis should be considered throughout the rest of the subjective and physical assessment, as well as during ongoing patient management.[3]

Initial clues can be gleaned from simple observation. Static observation of the equine athlete involves noting the conformation of the horse and comparing this with other horses of its breed. Mentation of the animal, as well as condition and muscular coverage for its age, type and level of work should be noted. Symmetry of musculature and bony landmarks, as well as weight bearing ability, may be compared from side to side. Occasionally anomalies that seem to be an asymmetry are not so; for example, a subtle shift in weight bearing through the forelimbs can make one side of the pectoral muscles seem larger than the other. This is where, further to static observation, movement assessment and palpation become an essential part of the physiotherapy examination.

Before palpation of the equine athlete, it is useful to gather further information about the presenting problem by watching the horse move. From the observation, the physiotherapist can determine the horse's willingness to move. If the horse has a frank lameness that had been undiagnosed, the horse should be returned to the veterinarian for a diagnosis. However, in most cases requiring a physiotherapy assessment, the horse may not be lame but may instead have a movement dysfunction or impairment. Basic walk or trot in a straight line may not highlight the impairment fully; thus, the physiotherapist may need to observe the horse performing a provoking activity.

A provoking activity or gait can be considered the functional assessment. Functional assessment is used in many areas of physiotherapy, including sports injury, and physiotherapists have moderate levels of reliability when using functional screening methods.[4] Functional assessment may include looking at whole gait or movements or dissecting out components of whole movements to see what the athlete can achieve in assessment. An example of a functional assessment for a human athlete is the weight bearing ankle dorsiflexion test.[5] This test shows consistent results between 1 or 2 testers. In the equine athlete, observation of various gaits on a small circle or hill, or working on soft surfaces over poles, or with rider in situ, are whole movement functional tests. **Fig. 1** demonstrates a horse walking uphill over spaced poles.

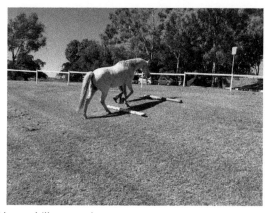

Fig. 1. Horse walking uphill over poles.

An example of a functional test as a component of another movement in the equine athlete is the ability of the horse to perform a "rounding reflex," which is a reflex motion to palpatory pressure. The rounding reflex demonstrates the ability of the horse to use the pelvic, abdominal, and back musculature to rotate the pelvis caudally and simultaneously flex through the thoracolumbar spine, an essential component of many equestrian sports. **Fig. 2** shows assessment of a horse's ability to cross the front limbs; this may be functional for a dressage movement. Another simple functional test is shown in **Fig. 3**. This is a baited stretch into left lateral cervical flexion. All these functional test can be used as interventions, as well as in reassessment.

The physiotherapist is directed toward the likely source of the impairment or movement dysfunction from the dynamic observation and functional testing. Enhancing the accuracy of physiotherapy diagnosis involves a combination of gathering information from the observation, and the clinical findings derived from palpatory examination.

The Physical Examination

This list, adapted from Goff,[1] outlines further stages of the physical physiotherapy examination, after the functional assessment:

- Active physiological movements;
- Soft tissues—palpation and testing;
- Passive physiological joint assessment;
- Passive accessory joint assessment; and

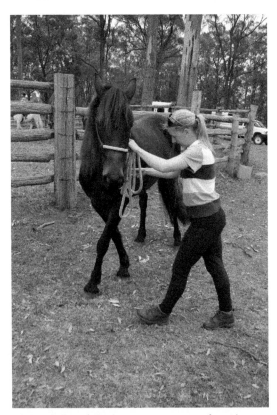

Fig. 2. Assessment of the ability of the horse to cross over front legs.

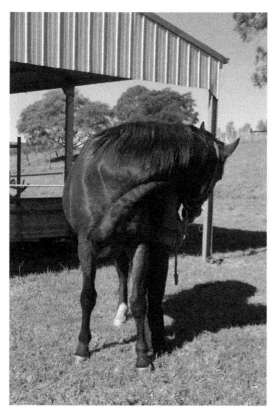

Fig. 3. Functional test of left lateral flexion (baited stretch).

- Neuromechanical tissue testing.

Active physiological movements can be grouped into functional assessments. They reveal what the equine athlete can achieve, and certainly which components of functional movements they cannot achieve.

Further, the physical examination is aimed at confirming the hypotheses and ideas suggested by the history and observation.[6,7] This confirmation is achieved from this point of the physiotherapy assessment of the equine athlete, by skilled and careful palpation. Physiotherapists devote much of their undergraduate degree time to training in palpation. Physiotherapists who then gain further experience or postgraduate training in the fields of manual or musculoskeletal physiotherapy and sports physiotherapy are well-prepared to conduct a skilled palpation of the musculoskeletal system of the horse. In human musculoskeletal medicine, physiotherapists now also use objective assessment tools such as real-time ultrasonography[8] to observe status of soft tissue injuries and motor control (See McGowan, Cottrial: Introduction to equine physical therapy and rehabilitation, in this issue). Palpation, however, remains a skill that is very important for gathering clinical information, although it is still considered among researchers to be subjective.[9–11]

Soft Tissue Palpation

Physiotherapists are trained to palpate the soft tissue system as well as the articular system. Because the articular structures are covered by extensive soft tissue (muscle, fascia, and neural tissue), it makes sense to perform palpation of the soft tissues initially. Goff[1] divides soft tissue palpation into general and specific. General soft tissue palpation provides the physiotherapist with information regarding temperature, soft tissue irritability, muscle tone, soft tissue thickening or swelling, and overall reactivity of the equine athlete to manual touch. General palpation is also an important part of the physiotherapist's communication with the animal patient, as a precedent to deeper palpation and further manual examination.

Muscles can be a primary source of pain and can be palpated for reactivity, as well as the parameters mentioned. Myofascial trigger points are promoted as an important cause of musculoskeletal pain, with many practitioners identifying myofascial trigger points.[12] These trigger points have been identified in horses, albeit in an observational study.[13] Despite a small number of studies showing that myofascial trigger point palpation in people is reliable,[14] systematic reviews reveal there is no accepted reference standard for the diagnosis of trigger points, and data on the reliability of physical examination for trigger points are conflicting.[12,15]

Thus, muscle palpation is a subjective assessment technique based on the physiotherapist's experience in feeling the quality of soft tissue. Algometry is a tool that can be used to more objectively measure muscle mechanical nociceptive threshold[16] and has been used in both human and animal research.[16–18] Algometry has been shown to be a repeatable modality for physiotherapy assessment of the horse,[19] and can be used in baseline assessment as well as reassessment (**Fig. 4**).

Specific muscle palpation should be carried out when the working hypothesis has caused the physiotherapist to believe that groups or individual muscles are a primary source of symptoms.[1] It is, therefore, necessary to develop a feel for variations in tone of musculature between different breeds and also states of arousal of horses. The physiotherapist should be able to differentiate between variations in muscle texture or tone. Alteration in muscle texture may manifest as general hypertonicity and hypotonicity, acute spasm, "boggy" (edematous), woody, or fibrous. Occasionally, the fascia covering the muscle group is not continuous. This may represent a recent or chronic fascial or muscle disruption.[1] Specific soft tissue palpation can also divulge the presence of scar tissue, effusions, or edema.

There are no strict guidelines for how to palpate the soft tissue of the equine athlete. The area of the horse's body often dictates the choice of the palpation technique. The primary goal of soft tissue palpation is to gather information. Manual therapists gather this information via the mechanoreceptors in the palmar surface of the hand and digits.[20] Hand contact must be kept firm, yet not be ticklish for the horse, "pokey,"

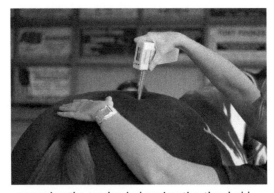

Fig. 4. Algometry—measuring the mechanical nociceptive threshold.

or harsh. The hand or hands of the physiotherapist should be relatively relaxed. Although there is evidence to suggest that the density of the mechanoreceptors in the human hand are greatest in the index and third finger, and more concentrated in the distal part of the digits,[20] the horse is generally more comfortable with the palpation technique if there is reasonable contact area of the hand or hands. Thus, when starting out as equine physiotherapists, palpation with the flat of the hand, keeping fingers "soft," is generally a technique that is quite acceptable to the horse. As the physiotherapist becomes more experienced, modification of palpation techniques may occur.

Palpation assessment techniques can be quite deep, yet remain comfortable for the horse if the palpation is appropriate. Palpation may be along, or across the direction of the muscle fibers. Speed of application of palpation also affects the reactivity of the horse, as well as how the practitioner perceives information.[20] Many 'lay practitioners' or technicians, apply a rapid palpatory force to the epaxial musculature of the equine athlete and claim that the horse is "sore" owing to the reflex motion to palpatory pressure created by the rapid delivery of technique. The same area may be palpated with more care, in the same environment, and not produce such a response. Indeed, a more careful palpation will provide the practitioner with more information about tissue quality and reactivity than a scant, quick palpation. Positioning the horse's body segments may also allow the physiotherapist to gather more information about a particular muscle, group of muscles, or fascia. Using the example of palpation of the brachiocephalicus muscle, the horse's neck is flexed laterally toward the physiotherapist, reducing tension in the brachiocephalicus muscle, allowing the physiotherapist to literally attain a good grasp of the muscle in question (**Fig. 5**).

A sound knowledge of the anatomy of the equine musculature allows the physiotherapist to identify which muscles are part of the symptom production or impairment. In addition, a side-to-side comparison of findings of specific muscle palpation can help to identify problem areas. It is then part of the clinical reasoning process to

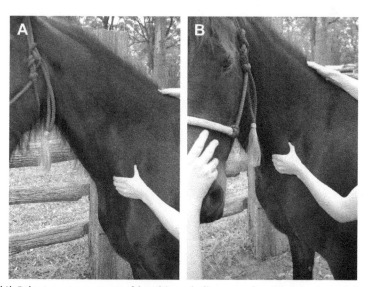

Fig. 5. (*A*) Palpatory assessment of brachiocephalicus muscle with horse's neck in neutral flexion. (*B*) Palpatory assessment of brachiocephalicus muscle with horse's neck in slight left lateral flexion.

determine if the findings are relevant to the clinical picture. Sometimes, the equine athlete is tender or "reactive" in certain muscle groups as a secondary compensation to another injury elsewhere, or factors such as poor saddle fit.

Physiotherapists are often involved in the rehabilitation of orthopedic conditions in the equine athlete, and thus must be able to assess the status of injured soft tissue to ascertain a base level of the injury at the commencement of physiotherapy intervention. One of the most common orthopedic injuries, tendinopathy of the superficial digital flexor tendon, involves adaptive changes within the tendon that are degenerative in nature.[21] The condition is diagnosed by ultrasound, and is characterized by thickening of the tendon similar to that of Achilles tendinopathy in people, and readily palpated. Serial ultrasound scans can determine the status of the tendon throughout rehabilitation; however, manual palpation gives the physiotherapist information regarding pain response and area of the tendon thickening as rehabilitation progresses.

Palpation of Peripheral Articular Structures

Equine physiotherapists should be skilled at palpating and moving the joints of the periphery and the vertebral column, including the temporomandibular joint, the pelvis and sacroiliac joint, and caudal vertebral joints. Examination of the peripheral joints involves the physiotherapist understanding the anatomy of the given joint and noting the presence of swelling, heat, ligament or capsular changes, and pain response of the horse when the soft tissues around joint are palpated. Palpation of the osseous architecture of the joint will also provide the physiotherapist with information about the clarity of the joint margins and bony proliferation. Further examination of the joint involves applying passive movement to the articulation and moving it throughout the readily available or physiological range. **Fig. 6** shows example of metacarpophalangeal joint full passive flexion. This maneuver is termed a passive physiological assessment of the joint and can be described as an osteokinematic movement. Knowledge of the kinematics of the horse's articular system is essential when assessing passive physiological movement of the peripheral joints. The physiotherapist notes the range of motion, the quality of the motion, and the end-feel. The range of motion can be compared with the same joint of the other side, or measured using objective tools, for example, goniometry[22] (**Fig. 7**). Ascertaining the quality of the movement refers to a more subjective assessment of whether there is crepitus present or if the joint motion is consistent and smooth throughout the range. Likewise, the end-feel of the joint may be recorded in descriptive terms, such as bony, soft, or springy. Experience will assist the physiotherapist in determining if the range and quality of the joint motion is

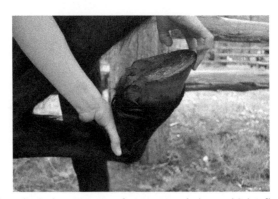

Fig. 6. Passive physiological assessment of metacarpophalangeal joint flexion.

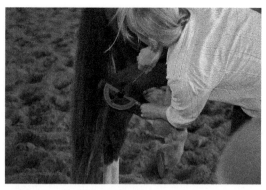

Fig. 7. Goniometry measurement of hock flexion.

significant in the clinical picture of movement dysfunction in the equine athlete. It is always useful to compare findings to the joint of the other side, especially when unsure as to the subjective findings.

Passive joint movement tests of the periphery can be taken further into passive accessory, or "translatory joint movements." If the physiotherapy assessment of the articular structure reveals a clinically relevant finding via passive physiological motion testing, the joint can be examined further using passive accessory testing. Passive accessory testing involves assessment of the motion between the joint surfaces applied to the joint by the therapist.[23] To apply the articular glides close to the joint margins, knowledge of the anatomy of the joint is essential. These articular glides provide the physiotherapist with information regarding the degree of accessory movement available at the joint, that is, whether the joint is hypermobile or hypomobile, or within normal limits, and also the end-feel of the joint. End-feel is described in a paper by Riddle[23] as bony, capsular, empty, springy, and spasm. End-feel is certainly subjective, and accessory glides or translatory movements are more difficult to measure than the osteokinematic passive physiological movements.

It is useful to keep in mind that when assessing articular structures, the passive joint motion tested affects intraarticular and periarticular structures (joint surfaces, joint capsule, ligaments) and to an extent also affects extraarticular structures, including musculature, fascia, and neuromeningeal tissue.[24] Because the horse has a large powerful musculature, and extensive layers of interconnected fascia, it is often easy for the practitioner to believe that the soft tissues are the most important tissue to address in assessment and treatment. However, the articular structures ultimately allow movement to occur at a given segment. Should there be reduced mobility, for example, in the case of osteoarthritis in the metacarpophalangeal joint, then treatment directed at the musculature of the shoulder and neck, which may be assessed as being reactive or reduced in length or normal tone in this case, will not be effective. Likewise, laxity or hypermobility of a joint can affect surrounding or related musculature as the equine athlete attempts to stabilize the segment or articulation during athletic performance. The related musculature may be assessed as reactive or hypertonic, and addressing this may not only be ineffective, but can lead to worsening of performance of the equine athlete. This highlights the importance of a thorough assessment of the musculoskeletal system, and also the importance of clinical reasoning.

Palpation of Articulations of the Vertebral Column

Hypermobility or hypomobility of joints occurs not only in the periphery, but also in the vertebral column of the equine athlete. Passive physiological and passive accessory articular assessment can be carried out at individual vertebral articulations, or in regions of the vertebral column. In functional assessment of the equine athlete, regions of the vertebral column rather than individual intervertebral segments are observed to be contributing to the overall movement. Unlike in the periphery, truly passive physiological intervertebral movement is more difficult to assess as the horse is standing while being examined and thus postural and trunk muscles are active. **Fig. 8** shows an example of the assessment of lateral flexion of the cervical spine. The physiotherapist can assess the amount of lateral flexion available at a given level of the cervical spine by localizing the lateral flexion to the chosen vertebral level, then applying a further translatory movement to the vertebrae. The end-feel and range of the translatory movement may be compared with other levels of the cervical spine or to the contralateral side. However, if there is excessive muscular activity owing to spasm or arousal of the horse, it is difficult to perform any type of passive articular assessment in the vertebral column. In more caudal regions of the vertebral column, it becomes a little more difficult to assess true intervertebral motion. This is where regions of the vertebral column are assessed. We know from human research that palpation of lumbar vertebral segments produces movements as far away as 3 vertebrae.[25] The speed and depth of application have also been suggested to affect

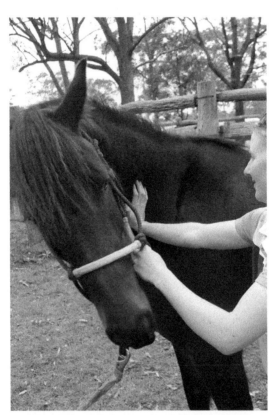

Fig. 8. Palpating the range of lateral flexion at a level of the cervical spine. This figure shows the right hand that is localizing, while the other hand induces the lateral flexion in the neck. The right hand of the physiotherapist applies a further translatory movement to the vertebrae.

intervertebral movement testing. Application of gentle dorsoventral force to a vertebral level, via the spinous process, would be less likely to influence adjacent vertebral segments than a vigorously applied force, and thus be more specific to the test segment.[20] **Fig. 9** shows a dorsoventrally directed manual palpation technique to a caudal lumbar vertebral segment.

In human manual therapy research, intersegmental spinal motion palpation has been shown to have low interrater reliability,[26] however, the intrarater reproducibility of manual spinal examination techniques is acceptable.[27,28] This does not mean that passive accessory and passive physiological testing of the vertebral column is not useful clinically, but that the quality of the research on interrater and intrarater reliability of spinal palpatory diagnostic procedures needs to be improved.[11] In human manual therapy, pain provocation techniques are the gold standard in manual testing of the vertebral column and sacroiliac joint. Pain provocation tests cannot be extrapolated to the equine athlete, because the tests require the subject to be able to verbalize the presence of pain. There has been comparatively very little research at all carried out into reliability of spinal motion palpation in the horse.

Passive physiological and passive accessory assessment can be performed for the sacroiliac region of the equine athlete. This is an important area to assess in the performance horse, because the forces from the large muscles of the pelvis and hindlimb are translated from the sacroiliac region to the trunk and further, cranially.[29] Relative motion between the ilium and the sacrum may be palpated during a physiological

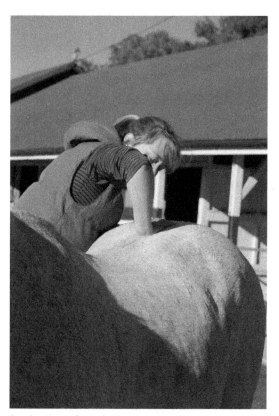

Fig. 9. Dorsoventral palpation of caudal lumbar vertebrae.

movement of full hind limb retraction or protraction. A dorsoventrally directed force over the tuber coxa of the horse produces the relative physiological motion of cranial rotation of the pelvis (**Fig. 10**). Accessory motion of the ilium relative to the sacrum may be palpated via a dorsoventrally directed glide onto the tubersacrale. Conversely, movement of the sacrum relative to the ilium may be assessed by applying a translatory force to the sacrum in a dorsoventral direction.

Neuromechanical Testing

Other tests that are used in the physiotherapy assessment of the equine athlete are tests of the status of the neural tissue and adjacent structures, specifically the ulnar, median, and radial nerves of the forelimb, and femoral and sciatic nerves in the hindlimb.[1] Neural provocation tests are used in human manual therapy to assess the effects on the neural tissue of the structures adjacent to the nervous system (the mechanical interface), and neurobiomechanics; that is, sliding of nerve alongside the interface and elongation. Neurodynamics are also affected by intraneural and extraneural edema and circulation.[24] Results from neural provocation testing may be sensitized by adding or removing a "central" component such as cervicothoracic or thoracolumbar flexion (equivalent to slump test in human physiotherapy).[30] The equine athlete cannot report reproduction of symptoms upon tensioning the neural tissue, so the physiotherapist must be sensitive to an increase in perceived tension of the

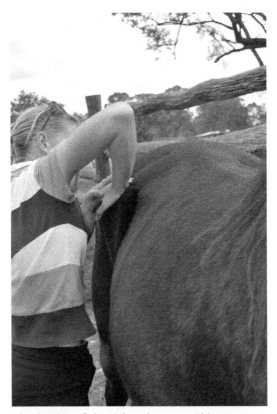

Fig. 10. Dorsoventral palpation of the right tuber coxa. This maneuver provides a relative cranial rotation of the right pelvis.

neuromeningeal structures, and should compare side to side. Neural provocations tests are used not only to establish the contribution of the structure to symptoms, but for reassessment and treatment. Babbage and colleagues[31] have documented testing of the canine sciatic nerve and its interfaces, but neuromechanical testing is not well-documented in horses. The equine "slump" test is an assessment that involves a tensioning or "winding up" of the spinal cord (via flexion of the trunk and neck) and adding tension to the sciatic nerve via protraction of the hind limb (**Fig. 11**). During assessment of the equine slump test, it may be more difficult to differentiate clearly between tension in the fascia and tension in neural tissue; sometimes these tissues are adjacent to and move with each other. Further research is required into this type of assessment.

OUTCOME MEASURES

Physiotherapists try, where possible, to use outcome measures in their assessment. This enables the equine physiotherapist to be more objective in their assessment when, as previously noted, much of the literature suggests that many of the manual tests that are carried out in musculoskeletal assessment have poor reliability. Standardized instruments for measuring patients' activity limitations and participation restrictions have been advocated for use by rehabilitation professionals for many years.[32] In physiotherapy practice, these instruments may include structured questionnaires, and measurement tools such as goniometers, tape measures, scales, and dynamometers. Photography and video are means by which to record baseline and then changes throughout assessment and treatment; many practitioners now carry smartphones and other devices that can readily record observable parameters.

In physiotherapy for the horse, goniometers, tape measures, and photography or video are used readily. Sometimes a handler is required to hold either the horse or body segments while the measurement is being carried out. **Figs. 12** and **13** show goniometry of the carpus and the metacarpophalangeal joint, respectively. **Fig. 14** shows measurement of cervical spine lateral bend, using a tape measure to a known bony landmark. **Fig. 15** shows the use of calipers to measure changes in swelling in a joint.

The use of such outcome measures by physiotherapists is important in the assessment of the equine athlete. Because there is little research regarding assessment

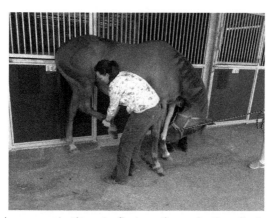

Fig. 11. Equine slump—cervicothoracic flexion, thoracolumbar flexion, and hind limb protraction.

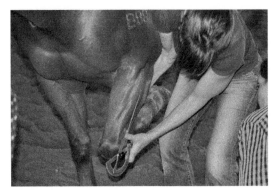

Fig. 12. Goniometry to measure carpal flexion.

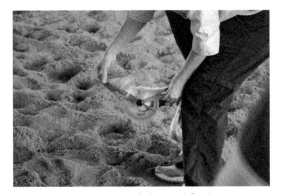

Fig. 13. Goniometry to measure metacarpophalangeal flexion.

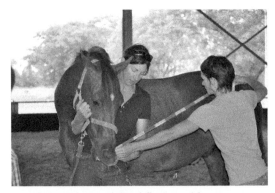

Fig. 14. Measurement of cervical spine lateral flexion with a tape measure.

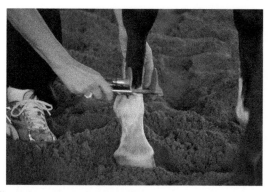

Fig. 15. Use of calipers to measure joint swelling.

techniques in the horse, physiotherapists can be accountable in the recording of baselines and changes that occur over time and during treatment.

SUMMARY

Equine physiotherapists use a functional approach to the assessment of the horse, compared with the traditional pathoanatomic diagnosis used by veterinarians. This enables equine physiotherapists to be consulted when there is a movement dysfunction, or poor performance, in the equine athlete. In this way, they work alongside and complement veterinary medicine. In the absence of good quality research into physiotherapy assessment techniques, equine physiotherapists try to use an evidence based approach to their assessment, which includes the use of outcome measures.

REFERENCES

1. Goff L. Physiotherapy assessment for animals. In: McGowan C, Goff L, editors. Animal physiotherapy – assessment, treatment and rehabilitation of animals. 2nd edition. John Wiley & sons Ltd; 2016. Chapter 11.
2. Adams C, Kurtz S. Coaching and feedback: enhancing communication teaching and learning in veterinary practice settings. J Vet Med Educ 2012;39:217–28.
3. Jones M. 1994, Clinical reasoning process in manipulative therapy. In: Boyling JD, Palastanga N, editors. Grieve's modern manual therapy, the vertebral column. 2nd edition. Edinburgh (United Kingdom): Churchill Livingstone; 1994. Chapter 34. p. 471–5.
4. Moran R, Schneiders A, Major K, et al. How reliable are functional movement screening scores? systematic review of rater reliability. Br J Sports Med 2015. [Epub ahead of print].
5. Powden C, Hoch J, Hoch M. Reliability and minimal detectable change of the weight-bearing lunge test: a systematic review. Man Ther 2015;20:524–32.
6. Refshauge K, Latimer J. The history. In: Refshauge K, Gass L, editors. Musculoskeletal physiotherapy – clinical science and practice. Oxford (United Kingdom): Butterworth Heinemann; 1995. p. 95, 111–5.
7. Refshauge K, Latimer J. The physical examination. In: Refshauge K, Gass L, editors. Musculoskeletal physiotherapy – clinical science and practice. Oxford (United Kingdom): Butterworth Heinemann; 1995. p. 95, 111–5.

8. Wallwork TL, Hides JA, Stanton WR. Intrarater and interrater reliability of assessment of lumbar multifidus muscle thickness using rehabilitative ultrasound imaging. J Orthop Sports Phys Ther 2007;37:608–12.

9. Van Trijffel E, Anderegg Q, Bossuyt P, et al. Inter-examiner reliability of passive assessment of intervertebral motion in the cervical and lumbar spine: a systematic review. Man Ther 2005;10:256–69.

10. Haneline M, Young MA. Review of intraexaminer and interexaminer reliability of static spinal palpation: a literature synthesis. J Ortho Manip Ther 2009;32:379–86.

11. Seffinger M, Najm W, Mishra S, et al. Reliability of spinal palpation for diagnosis of back and neck pain: a systematic review of the literature. Spine 2004;29: E413–25.

12. Lucas N, Macaskill P, Irwig L, et al. Reliability of physical examination for diagnosis of myofascial trigger points: a systematic review of the literature. Clin J Pain 2009;25:80–9.

13. Macgregor J, Graf von Schweinitz D. Needle electromyographic activity of myofascial trigger points and control sites in equine cleidobrachialis muscle–an observational study. Acupunct Med 2006;24:61–70.

14. Bron C, Franssen J, Wensing M, et al. Interrater reliability of palpation of myofascial trigger points in three shoulder muscles. J Man Manip Ther 2007;15:203–15.

15. Myburgh C, Holsgaard-Larsen A, Hartvigsen J. A systematic critical review of manual palpation for identifying myofascial trigger points: evidence and clinical significance. Arch Phys Med Rehabil 2008;89:1169–76.

16. Haussler K, Erb H. Mechanical nociceptive threshold in the axial skeleton of horses. Equine Vet J 2006;38:70–5.

17. Ohrbach R, Gale E. Pressure pain thresholds in normal muscles: reliability, measurement effects and topographic differences. Pain 1989;37:257–63.

18. Brown F, Robinson M, Riley J, et al. Better palpation of pain: reliability and validity of a new pressure pain protocol in TMD. Cranio 2000;18:58–65.

19. Varcoe-Cocks K, Sagar K, Jeffcott L, et al. Pressure algometry to quantify muscle pain in racehorses with suspected sacroiliac dysfunction. Equine Vet J 2006;38: 558–62.

20. Nyberg R, Russell Smith A. The science of spinal motion palpation: a review and update with implications for assessment and intervention. J Man Manip Ther 2013;21:160–7.

21. Patterson-Kane J, Firth E. Pathophysiology of exercise-induced superficial digital flexor tendon injury in thoroughbred racehorses. Vet J 2009;181:79–89.

22. Liljebrink Y, Bergh A. Goniometry: is it a reliable tool to monitor passive joint range of motion in horses? Equine Vet J Suppl 2010;38:676–82.

23. Riddle D. Measurement of accessory motion: critical issue and related concepts. Phys Ther 1992;72:865–74.

24. Coppieters M, Bartholomeeusen K, Stappaerts K. Incorporating nerve-gliding techniques in the conservative treatment of cubital tunnel syndrome. J Manipulative Physiol Ther 2004;27:560–8.

25. Lee R, Evans J. Load-displacement-time characteristics of the spine under posteroanterior mobilisation. Aust J Physiother 1992;38:115–23.

26. Haneline M, Cooperstein R, Young M, et al. Spinal motion palpation: a comparison of studies that assessed intersegmental end feel vs excursion. J Manipulative Physiol Ther 2008;31:616–26.

27. Stochkendahl M, Christensen H, Hartvigsen J, et al. Manual examination of the spine: a systematic critical literature review of reproducibility. J Manipulative Physiol Ther 2006;29:475–85.

28. Snodgrass S, Rivett D, Robertson V. Manual forces applied during cervical mobilization. J Manipulative Physiol Ther 2007;30:17–25.
29. Jeffcott L, Dalin G, Ekman S, et al. Sacroiliac lesions as a cause of chronic poor performance in competitive horses. Equine Vet J 1985;17:111–8.
30. Coppieters M, Butler D. In defense of neural mobilisation. J Orthop Sports Phys Ther 2001;31:520–1.
31. Babbage C, Coppieters M, McGowan C. Strain and excursion of the sciatic nerve in the dog: Biomechanical considerations in the development of a clinical test for increased neural mechanosensitivity. Vet J 2007;174:330–6.
32. Jette DU, Halbert J, Iverson C, et al. Use of standardized outcome measures in physical therapist practice: perceptions and applications. Phys Ther 2009;89: 125–35.

Core Training and Rehabilitation in Horses

Hilary M. Clayton, BVMS, PhD, MRCVS[a,b,*]

KEYWORDS

- Horse • Back pain • Core training • Dynamic mobilization exercises
- Balancing exercises

KEY POINTS

- The central body axis or core is a key component in controlling body posture and providing a stable platform for limb movements and generation of locomotor forces.
- The superficially located, mobilizing muscles control global movements of the spine and transmit locomotor forces from the limbs to the trunk.
- The deep stabilizing muscles have short fascicles that provide postural support, move localized areas of the spine, and provide spinal stability before and during locomotion.
- Persistent dysfunction of the deep stabilizing muscles seems to be common in horses indicating a need for core training exercises to restore normal function.
- It is recommended that core training be performed throughout the horse's athletic career to maintain a healthy back as well as used therapeutically when back pain is identified.

CORE ANATOMY, FUNCTION, AND DYSFUNCTION

The horse's body consists of a series of axial segments (the head, neck, and trunk) and the 4 limbs that support and move the entire body. The core is the axial skeleton together with the soft tissues that have their proximal attachment on the axial skeleton, which includes the spinal ligaments, epaxial and hypaxial musculature, together with the extrinsic limb musculature of the thoracic synsarcoses and the pelvic girdle that transfers locomotor forces generated by the limbs to the axial segments.

Based on the orientation of the articular facets Townsend and Leach[1] divided the thoracolumbosacral spine into 4 functional regions: T1-T2, T2-T16, T16-L6, and L6-S1. Movement at each intervertebral joint is small except at the extremities;

[a] Michigan State University, Department of Large Animal Clinical Sciences, 736 Wilson Road, East Lansing, MI 48824, USA; [b] Sport Horse Science, LLC, 3145 Sandhill Road, Mason, MI 48854, USA
* Michigan State University, Department of Large Animal Clinical Sciences, 736 Wilson Road, East Lansing, MI 48824.
E-mail address: claytonh@cvm.msu.edu

Vet Clin Equine 32 (2016) 49–71
http://dx.doi.org/10.1016/j.cveq.2015.12.009 **vetequine.theclinics.com**
0749-0739/16/$ – see front matter © 2016 Elsevier Inc. All rights reserved.

cranially the first thoracic (T1-T2) joint contributes to neck movements, and caudally the lumbosacral joint (L6-S1) allows pelvic tilting that contributes to protraction and retraction of the hind limbs.[1] Movement of these joints is facilitated by having wider intervertebral disks at T1-T2, T2-T3, and L6-S1 and restricted, in part, by the orientation of the articular facets.[1]

According to the bow and string model,[2] the equine thoracolumbar spine acts like a flexible bow that is maintained in a slightly arched (rounded) position by tension in the string, formed by the abdominal and sublumbar muscles. Concentric contraction of these muscles rounds the back by flexing the intervertebral joints. Insufficient tension in the string allows the weight of the viscera to extend the intervertebral joints, and the back contour becomes more lordotic. It is desirable for horses to work in a rounded posture to maintain separation of the dorsal spinous processes, so the use of conditioning exercises that recruit and strengthen the hypaxial musculature is an important part of athletic training. In horses that have poor natural posture or weak, inactive hypaxial muscles, for example, following colic surgery or foaling, the rehabilitation program should target activation and strengthening of these muscles. Appropriate exercises include core training from the ground as well as specific types of locomotor exercises.

The epaxial and hypaxial muscles have many similarities across species.[3,4] The long mobilizing muscles are located superficially, which increases their leverage at the intervertebral joints. They cross many vertebral levels and have a global effect on entire regions of the spine, but they cannot confine their action to a single joint or a localized area. The deep stabilizing muscles cross only one to a few intervertebral joints, which allows them to have a more localized effect that stabilizes individual joints or changes the shape of the neck or back in a specific area. They lie adjacent or very close to the vertebrae, so their moment arms are short, which gives them less leverage than the long mobilizers but facilitates their role in providing stabilization when the joints are loaded during locomotion.[3] Without this stability the joints undergo micromotion between the articulating surfaces during locomotion, which predisposes to the development of arthritic changes. A characteristic of the deep stabilizing muscles is that they have a lower activation threshold than the long mobilizing muscles,[5] so they are preactivated in preparation for locomotion. Consequently, the intervertebral joints are stabilized before the onset of an intentional movement or during a perturbation of movement.

The abdominal muscles surround the belly in layers. Their functions include dorsoventral flexion, lateral bending and stabilization of the back, respiration, support and protection of the viscera, and pressurization of the abdominal cavity, which also aids in stability. The two deepest layers, the transverse abdominal muscle and, to a lesser extent, the internal oblique muscle, function as deep spinal stabilizers and they are activated in anticipation of movement to provide proactive (feed forward) control of spinal stability.[5] In the standing horse, the transverse abdominal muscle shows low-amplitude tonic activity that increases in the terminal part of expiration, whereas the activity of the internal abdominal oblique varies between horses, with some showing tonic, low-amplitude activity unrelated to breathing, whereas others have phasic activity during the later stage of expiration.[6] In dogs it has been shown that the internal, but not the external, oblique muscles contribute to sagittal plane stabilization that opposes hollowing of the back, especially when extra weight is added to the midback.[7] The more superficial musculus (m) rectus abdominis and external abdominal oblique muscles are global mobilizers that contribute to flexion and lateral bending of the back. During quiet standing, m rectus abdominis shows either no activity or low-amplitude tonic activity.[7] The between-horse variability in activation of the abdominal muscles may indicate different postural control strategies.

The equine sublumbar muscles (m iliopsoas, m psoas minor) attach proximally to the underside of the last 3 thoracic vertebrae, the lumbar vertebrae, the sacrum, and the ilium, and run to the cranial aspect of the pelvis and femur. A high percentage of type I muscle fibers are present in m psoas minor, indicating a postural support function, whereas m iliopsoas has predominantly type IIX fibers that can actively flex the lumbosacral and hip joints.[8] Both of these actions protract the hind limbs and contribute to the horse's ability to work in collection. Not surprisingly, the sublumbar muscles can become tight in horses that perform a lot of collected work; these horses benefit from passive stretching of the hip joint in extension. This stretching can be achieved through retracting the hind limb by extending the hip joint and holding the stretch for about 30 seconds. The therapist should take care to perform this stretch with regard to personal safety and correct ergonomics (**Fig. 1**).

The epaxial musculature, located dorsal to the ribs or transverse processes on either side of the dorsal spinous processes (**Fig. 2**), is similar in structure and function across species.[3,4,9] In horses, the long mobilizing muscles, m longissimus dorsi and m iliocostalis, have a predominance of type IIX muscle fibers[8]; they cross many vertebral levels and have a global effect on the entire thoracolumbar spine. Simultaneous concentric contraction of the left and right muscles extends the intervertebral joints and hollows the back, whereas unilateral concentric contraction assists in lateral bending.[10–12] The m multifidi are deep stabilizing muscles located adjacent to the dorsal spinous processes. At each vertebral level, m multifidi have 5 fascicles arranged in layers. The short, overlapping, pennated fibers are separated and connected by fibrous tissue[13] and the deepest layers have the highest percentage of type I fibers[8] which are the shortest fibers spanning a single joint. These fibers oppose rotational

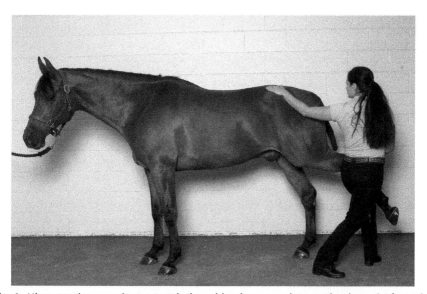

Fig. 1. Hip extension exercise to stretch the sublumbar musculature. The therapist faces the horse and retracts the distal hind limb by hooking the horse's tarsal joint over her own thigh. Retraction is increased as the muscles relax. The stretched position is held for at least 30 seconds. (*From* Stubbs NC, Clayton HM. Activate your horse's core. Mason (MI): Sport Horse Publications; 2008; with permission.)

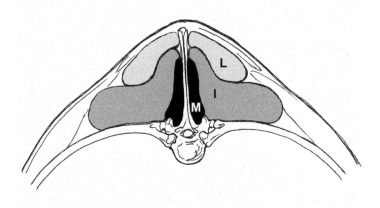

Fig. 2. Cross section through the withers showing the 3 epaxial muscles. I, m iliocostalis; L, m longissimus; M, m multifidi.

or shear forces generated by the transverse and oblique abdominal muscles in people[9,13] and seem to act similarly in horses.[3] The more superficial fascicles of m multifidi have longer moment arms at the intervertebral joints and fewer slow twitch fibers than the deeper fascicles[8]; they are thought to contribute both to stabilization and movement of the individual intervertebral joints that causes localized changes in shape of the spine.[3] The contribution of m multifidi to normal motion patterns was confirmed by showing that spinal kinematics changed after injecting local anesthetic solution into m multifidi of sound horses.[14] The action of the deep stabilizing muscles improves the quality of the horse's performance, especially in movements, such as flying changes or jumping, that require effective transmission of potentially destabilizing forces from the hind limbs.

Because m multifidi have a larger component of fibrous tissue than the surrounding muscles, it can be distinguished from them ultrasonographically, which allows its borders to be traced and its cross-sectional area (CSA) to be calculated (**Fig. 3**). A technique for measuring ultrasonographic CSA of the equine m multifidi in the thoracolumbar region has been described and shown to be reliable and repeatable.[13,15]

Back pain is common and often recurrent in people[16] and horses.[17–19] Because of the huge economic impact of low back pain in the human population, there has been considerable research into the function and dysfunction of the epaxial muscles; based on current evidence, horses seem to follow the same pattern of neuromotor dysfunction[15] and response to therapy.[20–22]

Although there are many inciting causes of back pain, they tend to follow a common pathway involving changes in neuromotor control and rapid (within days) neurogenic atrophy of m multifidi at the affected spinal level on the ipsilateral side.[23] Atrophy is selective for m multifidi and does not involve other epaxial muscles.[24] Inhibition of m multifidi allows spinal instability and micromotion of the intervertebral joints that predisposes to the development of further pathologies, such as osteoarthritis.[25] Unilateral atrophy of m multifidi results in significant left-right asymmetry in CSA with the smaller

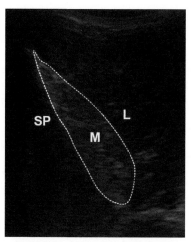

Fig. 3. Ultrasonographic image of the epaxial muscles at the level of T12 on the left side. The m multifidi, which appear whiter than m longissimus because of the greater content of fibrous tissue, are outlined by the white dashed line. L, m longissimus; M, m multifidi; SP, dorsal spinous process.

muscle located on the painful side.[26] Even after the initial episode of back pain resolves, m multifidi remain dysfunctional and atrophied, which increases the likelihood of a recurrence of back pain.[25] In an attempt to break this cycle, patients may perform specific motor control exercises that have been shown to reactivate and strengthen m multifidi[27] and reduce the risk of recurrence of back pain within the next 12 months from greater than 80% to around 30%.[28] Thus, physiotherapy is an efficient and cost-effective way both to treat and to prevent recurrence of back pain in people.

In horses, it has not yet been proven that back pain per se causes neurogenic atrophy of m multifidi, but severe vertebral osseous lesions have been associated with atrophy of m multifidi ipsilaterally at the same spinal level resulting in left-right asymmetry in CSA.[15] In an attempt to compensate for the inactivation of m multifidi, tension in m longissimus dorsi increases, causing palpable muscle spasms.[29,30] However, the architecture of m longissimus is not appropriate for stabilization of the individual intervertebral joints, instead tonic contraction causes general stiffness of the horse's back and movements. Both spinal (McTimoney) manipulations and reflex inhibition therapy have been shown to reduce muscle tone in m longissimus.[11]

In accordance with the human back pain model, it is reasonable to hypothesize that m multifidi will not resume normal activity spontaneously, even after the cause of inactivation resolves. Therefore, physiotherapeutic exercises that target m multifidi may be needed to reactivate and strengthen these muscles in horses that have had back pain, especially if the CSA of m multifidi is asymmetrical on the left and right sides. Evidence-based research has shown that dynamic mobilization exercises (DMEs) are effective for this purpose,[20–22] and there are anecdotal reports that other core strengthening exercises may also be useful.

The extrinsic muscles of the limbs are included as part of the core because they determine how effectively forces are transmitted from the limbs to the trunk; their activity is essential for maintaining the horse's balance, especially when perturbations are applied to the body. The pelvic stabilizer muscles control pelvic alignment and movements when the hind limb is grounded. The gluteal and hamstring muscles, especially m biceps femoris, which crosses the lateral aspect of the hip joint, maintain the alignment of the femur and pelvis. In the forelimb the thoracic sling muscles suspend the ribcage between the forelimbs in the standing horse. During locomotion, coordinated activity in the left and right sling muscles is necessary to maintain elevation of the forehand (self-carriage) and prevent the shoulders leaning into or out of the turns. Most of the forelimb extrinsic muscles (pectorals, m latissimus dorsi, m subclavius, m trapezius and m rhomboideus) have long fascicles arranged in parallel with the long axis of the muscle, which is typical of muscles that contract through a large range of motion. M serratus ventralis thoracis differs from the other extrinsic muscles in having short, highly pennated fascicles, consistent with an antigravitational role; its muscle belly is sandwiched between 2 broad, thick aponeurotic sheets that contribute to the elastic properties of the forelimb.[31] In the standing horse m serratus ventralis shows marked tonic activity consistent with providing postural support and stabilization for the chest.[6]

EFFECT OF THE RIDER ON SPINAL POSTURE AND MOVEMENT

Posture refers to the position of the body parts and the overall effect on the horse's carriage. When the body segments are correctly aligned, it reduces the energy expended to maintain the body's position during standing and locomotion. In horses, good posture includes rounding the back and lifting through the withers (**Fig. 4**). The equine thoracolumbar spine, supported cranially by the forelimbs and caudally by the hind limbs, tends to sag in the middle, pulled down by the considerable weight of the viscera. When the additional weight of a rider is added to the horse's back,

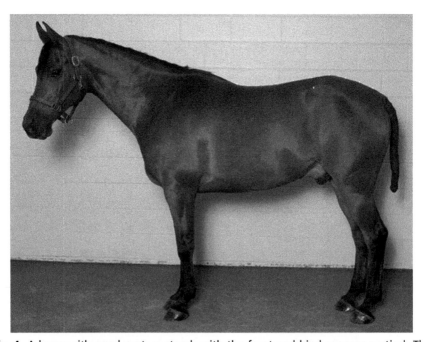

Fig. 4. A horse with good posture stands with the front and hind cannons vertical. The topline shows elevation of the withers, limited lordosis of the midthoracic region, and a smooth well-muscled coupling over the loin to the croup. The abdominal musculature is taut.

thoracolumbar lordosis increases both at stance and during locomotion.[32] During locomotion the range of back motion during a stride does not change but the entire motion cycle is more extended compared with the unridden horse. One of the undesirable effects of extension of the intervertebral joints is that it approximates the dorsal spinal processes, so it is not surprising that impingement and overriding of the dorsal spinous processes occur most frequently and are most severe in the mid to caudal thoracic region,[19,22] which is the area directly below the rider's seat. The likelihood of developing clinical signs associated with impingement is ameliorated when intervertebral extension is reduced.

PRINCIPLES OF REHABILITATION FOR THE CORE MUSCULATURE

Reactivation of m multifidi is an important component of rehabilitation in horses with back pain. In people, therapeutic exercises are used to enhance motor learning and stimulate cocontraction of the deep stabilizing muscles (m transversus abdominis and m multifidi).[33] The most successful exercises for restoring function of m multifidi combine stabilization training with an alternation between static and dynamic muscular activity. Incorporation of a static holding component between the concentric and eccentric phases seems to be particularly beneficial.[24] It is more effective to enhance motor patterns that stimulate many muscles rather than trying to target a single muscle.[27]

In horses, core training exercises are intended to activate and strengthen not only the epaxial muscles but also the abdominal and sublumbar muscles that are so important for good posture. Evidence-based studies have shown that DMEs (baited stretches) increase the CSA of m multifidi.[20–22] The term *dynamic* indicates that the horse's musculature is actively moving the body, and *mobilization* implies that the joints are being moved through their full range of motion. However, the main benefit of these exercises lies in their ability to activate and strengthen the muscles that stabilize the spine rather than for enhancing flexibility. The use of techniques to activate the deep stabilizing muscles is in accordance with motor control principles indicating that it is more important to restore stability and muscular strength than to increase flexibility.

DYNAMIC MOBILIZATION EXERCISES

Dynamic spinal mobilization is achieved when the horse follows a controlled movement pattern that recruits both the long mobilizing muscles and the deep stabilizing muscles to round or bend the neck and back. The horse is taught to follow a controlled movement pattern using a bait, such as a piece of carrot or a target through a specific movement pattern that involves rounding and/or lateral bending of the neck and back while stabilizing the back and limbs to maintain balance. A large number of muscles are recruited, including the abdominal, epaxial, pelvic, hamstring, and pectoral muscles. Initially, the horse should be taught the exercises while standing in a square and balanced position; but horses that are familiar with the exercises can be challenged by performing them in a variety of stance positions, with a leg raised or on unstable surfaces. The optimal time to perform DMEs is immediately before exercise each day to preactivate the postural control muscles.

Carrots cut lengthways into pieces about 1 cm in diameter work well as bait. It is recommended that leather gloves be worn as finger protection when using bait. An alternative is to use target training with a clicker to signal the correct response. When teaching the horse to perform DMEs, it is useful to have a second person to steady the haunches. If a helper is not available, the horse can be backed into a corner or positioned against a wall to discourage limb movements and teach the horse to follow the bait by moving the head and neck without swinging the haunches in the opposite direction. In the beginning, a small amount of movement is rewarded. Over a period of several days, the demands are gradually increased until the desired position or the end range of motion has been reached. The horse is encouraged to hold the position for several seconds, and it is sometimes helpful to use the free hand to stabilize the horse in the desired position. After each attempt, allow the muscles to relax for several seconds. Perform 3 to 5 repetitions of each exercise per day; for the lateral bending exercises, do an equal number of repetitions to the left and right sides.[34]

Rounding Exercises

Rounding exercises flex the intervertebral joints as the horse follows the bait to specific positions on the ventral midline (**Fig. 5**). The neck should remain straight without any twisting motion. Straightness can be encouraged by standing alternately on the left and right sides while performing the mobilizations or by having an assistant hold the noseband to stabilize the head on the midline. The muscles in different parts of the neck and back are stimulated in different rounding positions. The following series of rounding exercises may be performed with intervertebral angular changes as described by Clayton and colleagues[35]:

- Chin to mid-neck: The poll is maximally flexed as the chin moves close to the underside of the neck.
- Chin to chest: The poll is highly flexed as the chin moves to the level of the manubrium.
- Chin between carpi: The chin moves caudally between the carpi rounding the base of the neck and cranial thoracic regions but with less flexion at the poll.

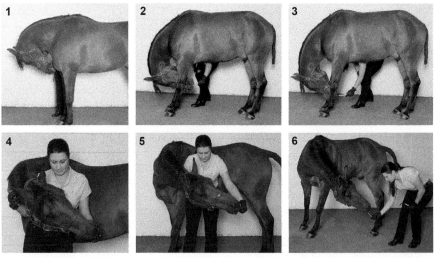

Fig. 5. Examples of DMEs. 1, chin-to-chest rounding; 2, chin-between-knees rounding; 3, chin-between-fore-fetlocks rounding; 4, chin-to-girth bending; 5, chin-to-flank bending; 6, chin-to-hind-fetlock bending. When the chin is moved between the carpi or fetlocks, the limbs must be separated sufficiently for the horse's head to pass between them. Some horses, especially those with short necks, flex their carpi when reaching deeply down and back; but this is not a problem so long as the neck is fully flexed. (*From* Stubbs NC, Clayton HM. Activate your horse's core. Mason (MI): Sport Horse Publications; 2008; with permission.)

- Chin between fetlocks: The chin moves ventrally between the front fetlocks by flexing at the base the neck and in the thoracic region while extending the angle at the poll.

Lateral Bending Exercises

Lateral bending exercises move the head and neck laterally (see **Fig. 5**) and, of course, are performed equally to the left and right sides while observing for any asymmetry in range of motion between the two sides. Twisting of the neck should be discouraged; ideally the two ears should stay at the same height. If necessary, the therapist's free arm can be used to discourage head twisting. The chin can be moved to a variety of positions while the therapist observes the effect on spinal motion, which varies between horses. In an individual horse, exercises that hollow the back should be avoided. Intervertebral angles during performance of lateral bending exercises have been described[36]:

- Chin to point of shoulder: The poll is maximally bent laterally. The free hand can be placed against the outside of the neck to help maintain the position for several seconds.
- Chin to girth: The chin moves to a position about 1 m lateral to the girth line. The therapist can stand inside the curve of the neck to encourage some bending in the midneck.
- Chin to flank: The chin moves to a position about 1 m lateral to the flank. Most of the bending occurs around the cervicothoracic junction with the thoracic spine also showing some flexion and lateral bending.
- Chin to hind fetlock: The chin moves caudoventrally to end range of motion with maximal lateral bending at the base of the neck while the joints in the upper neck are counterbent. The thoracic spine flexes and bends laterally. Because this mobilization approaches the end range of motion, it is likely that the horse will be able to reach progressively further over time.

Neck Extension Exercise

The horse stretches the neck forward in a low position as an unwinding exercise after performing the rounding and bending mobilizations. When teaching the neck extension exercise, it is helpful to have a low barrier, such as a stall guard, across the horse's chest to prevent stepping forward. The head should reach as far forward as possible, extending and stretching the cervical intervertebral joints.

Evidence-Based Research on Dynamic Mobilization Exercises

Kinematic studies have shown that during the performance of DMEs, most of the intervertebral motion involves the joints at the base of the neck (C5 to T1), which are used to flex, extend, and bend the entire neck, and the joints in the poll region (occiput to C2) that adjust the position of the head and vestibular organs. At the same time, the horse must also stabilize the back and limb girdles using the deep stabilizing musculature, which is a key benefit of these exercises. Three studies, each involving a different population of horses, have confirmed that DMEs stimulate hypertrophy of m multifidi.

In the first study, Stubbs and colleagues[22] used 8 riding school horses. They performed a series of DMEs consisting of 3 rounding exercises (chin to chest, chin between carpi, chin between fetlocks), 3 lateral bending exercises (chin to girth, chin to hip, chin to hind fetlock) performed to the left and right sides, and a neck extension exercise. Five repetitions of each exercise were performed daily on 5 days per week for 12 weeks during which time the horses were stabled overnight, turned out in small paddocks during the day, and did not receive any additional exercise. The CSA of m multifidi was measured at the start and end of the study on the left and right sides at 6 vertebral levels: T10, T12, T14, T16, T18, and L5. Statistical analysis showed that the muscular CSA increased significantly at every spinal level on both the left and right sides (**Fig. 6**). Furthermore, there was a significant reduction in asymmetry between the CSA of the left and right m multifidi at all 6 spinal levels. This study showed that regular performance of DMEs for 12 weeks stimulated significant hypertrophy of m multifidi in horses that were on the equivalent of bed rest.

In the second study,[20] 9 therapeutic riding horses were assigned to one of 3 groups, all of which continued their normal exercise regime throughout the study. This regime consisted of giving lessons of 25-minute duration 3 times per week on alternate days. The first group received no additional exercise; the other 2 groups performed the same series of DMEs that were used in the study of Stubbs and colleagues,[22] but the exercises were performed on only 3 days per week for 6 weeks. The third group of horses additionally performed a series of gymnastic exercises aimed specifically at recruiting and strengthening the abdominal and pelvic stabilizer muscles with the goal of increasing stride length, which is thought to improve the quality of the therapeutic riding experience. The gymnastic exercises were pelvic tilting, backing up, making tight turns around a barrel, and walking over a raised pole. They were performed on 3 days per week for 6 weeks. CSA of m multifidi, measured ultrasonographically at the level of L6, increased significantly ($P<.05$) in both groups that performed DMEs (**Fig. 7**). This study built on the findings of Stubbs and colleagues[22] in which the exercises were performed 5 days per week for 12 weeks by showing that an equivalent effect on m multifidi CSA was achieved by performing DMEs only 3 times per week for 6 weeks. It is evident from **Fig. 7** that the horses studied by de Oliviera and colleagues[20] initially had a smaller CSA than those studied by Stubbs and colleagues[22] and increased by a larger amount to reach approximately the same final CSA in both studies.

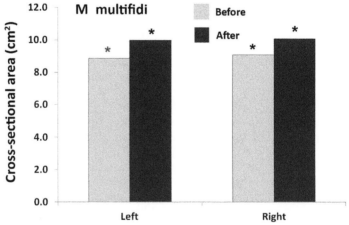

Fig. 6. Ultrasonographic CSA of m multifidi (N = 8) measured on the left and right sides before and after performing a series of dynamic mobilization exercises (DME) on 5 days per week for 12 weeks. Each value is averaged over 6 spinal levels (T10, T12, T14, T16, T18, L5). Asterisks indicate pairs of values that differ significantly ($P<.05$). (*Data from* Stubbs NC, Kaiser LJ, Hauptman J, et al. Dynamic mobilization exercises increase cross sectional area of musculus multifidus. Equine Vet J 2011;43:522–9.)

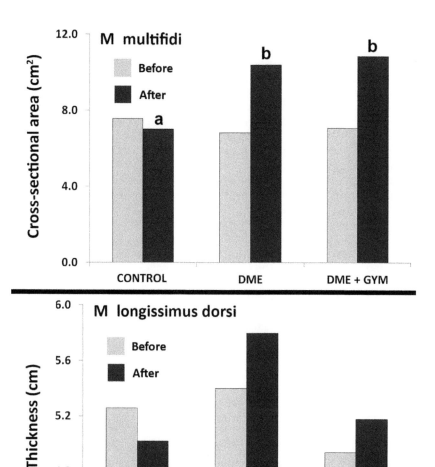

Fig. 7. Ultrasonographic CSA of m multifidi measured on the left side at L6' (*above*) and thickness of m longissimus measured on the left side at the level of the 17th to 18th ribs (*below*) at the start and end of the study. All horses performed 25-minute therapeutic riding lessons on 3 (alternate) days per week over the 6-week period of study. The control group (N = 3) was otherwise sedentary with no additional exercise. The second group (DME, N = 3) performed DMEs 3 days per week. The third group (DME + GYM, N = 3) performed both DMEs and a series of gymnastic exercises 3 days per week. Different letters above the columns indicate significant differences between treatment groups at the end of the study (*P*<.05). (*Data from* de Oliveira K, Soutello RVG, da Fonseca R, et al. Gymnastic training and dynamic mobilization exercises improve stride quality and epaxial muscle size in therapy horses. J Equine Vet Sci 2015;35:888–93.)

This study also measured the thickness of m longissimus dorsi at the level of the last 2 ribs and found that it increased in both groups that performed additional gymnastic exercises, but the difference did not reach statistical significance in either group (see **Fig. 7**). It should be noted that the gymnastic exercises were performed at walk because this is the working gait of the therapy horses; inclusion of trot or canter may have been more effective because activation of m longissimus is greater at trot than at walk.[12,37] Horses that performed the gymnastic exercises showed significant increases in stride length and tracking length when walking at the same speed before and after the exercise program,[20] which was regarded as a specific beneficial effect for therapy horses.

The third study involved a more athletic population of thoroughbred racehorses in training in the United Kingdom.[21] The 12 horses in the study were randomly divided into 2 groups; both groups continued their normal race training program, and the intervention group also performed the series of DMEs as described by Stubbs and colleagues[22] with 10 repetitions per day on 5 days per week for 12 weeks. CSA of m multifidi was measured at T16 on the left and right sides at the start of the study, after 6 weeks and after 12 weeks. The CSA of m multifidi did not change in the control group; but in the group performing DMEs, there was a significant increase in CSA after performing the exercises for 6 weeks and then no further increase at 12 weeks (**Fig. 8**).

Based on these 3 studies, it is concluded that performing 5 repetitions of each mobilization 3 times per week for as little as 6 weeks stimulates significant hypertrophy of

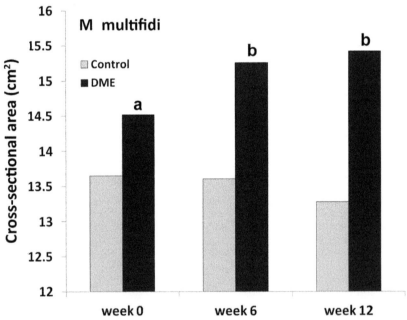

Fig. 8. Ultrasonographic CSA of m multifidi measured on the left and right sides at the level of T16 at the start and at 6 weekly intervals. The control group (N = 6) continued in race training. The second group (N = 6) continued in race training and also performed a series of DMEs 5 days per week for 12 weeks. Different letters above the columns indicate significantly different values within a treatment group at the 3 evaluations ($P<.05$). (*Data from* Tabor G. The effect of dynamic mobilisation exercises on the equine multifidus muscle and thoracic profile. [MS thesis]. Plymouth, UK: Plymouth University; 2015.)

m multifidi and there does not seem to be additional benefits from performing a larger number of repetitions or doing the exercises more frequently. It is recommended that this regimen be used in young horses to activate and strengthen the core musculature in preparation for ridden exercise. Regular performance of the exercises should be continued throughout the horse's athletic career to maintain preactivation of the deep stabilizing musculature. DMEs are also useful if a horse is on stall rest because of illness or injury and during rehabilitation from colic surgery when it is recommended that the exercises begin 1 month after surgery if there are no complications with wound healing.

CORE STRENGTHENING EXERCISES

Core strengthening exercises[38] are regarded as a progression from the DMEs. They address the postural muscles that affect the horse's balance and self-carriage and are particularly valuable in horses with a hollow topline or sagging abdomen. The exercises are based on the horse's response to pressure applied to specific anatomic areas. Some therapists apply pressure with their fingers, and others prefer to use a blunt tool. The pressure is perceived as a mildly noxious stimulus to which the horse responds by flexion and/or lateral bending of specific intervertebral joints through activation of the long mobilizing muscles in the cervical, thoracic, or lumbar regions. Electromyographic studies have shown that m longissimus dorsi is activated during stimulated extension or lateral bending of the thoracolumbar spine with activity being greater at T12 than at T16 or L3.[39] It is likely that the deep stabilizing muscles are also recruited, though this has not yet been proven in horses. The position can be held for several seconds by maintaining the stimulus. After each exercise, the muscles are allowed to relax for a few seconds before repeating. It is recommended that 3 to 5 repetitions of each technique be performed on several days per week. As with the DMEs, the most effective time to use core strengthening exercises is immediately before exercise to preactivate the muscles that will round and stabilize the spine during athletic activity.

Sternum, Withers, and Thoracic Lifting

The therapist stands facing the horse's shoulder and passes the hand closer to the horse's tail between the forelimbs. Upward pressure is applied over the sternum on the ventral midline starting between the pectoral muscles and slowly moving caudally between the forelimbs and beyond the girth line while maintaining a steady pressure. The horse responds by lifting sequentially through the base of the neck, the withers, and the cranial thoracic region. The raised position should be maintained by continuing to apply pressure for about 5 seconds. Some horses respond nicely to a scratching motion in the girth region that can be applied with the fingers, a blunt tool, or even a currycomb.

Lateral Lifting at the Withers

The therapist stands facing the withers and reaches across the ventral midline in the girth region with one hand. Pressure is applied starting 10 to 20 cm beyond the midline and moving slowly toward the midline. The horse responds by raising the withers laterally toward the therapist.

Lumbar and Lumbosacral Lifting

Pressure on the dorsal midline above the tail head or in the intermuscular groove between m biceps femoris and m semitendinosus stimulates the abdominal and sublumbar muscles to contract. This has the effect of lifting the lumbar region, flexing the lumbosacral joint, and tilting the pelvis caudally which have the effect of rounding the caudal part of the back. In the first technique, firm pressure is applied to the dorsal spinous processes starting at the tail head and moving cranially, one spine at a time, until the horse responds. The second technique involves stroking ventrally in the intermuscular furrow while applying just enough pressure to stimulate a slow, smooth rounding. Applying too much pressure or moving the hands too rapidly causes an abrupt, jerky response that is less desirable. If pressure is maintained, the position can be held for a few seconds before removing the pressure and allowing the back to return to the resting position.

Lumbar Lifting and Lateral Bending

Pressure lateral to the midline in the lumbar region stimulates lifting and lateral bending of the horse's pelvic region. The therapist reaches across the top of the haunches then applies pressure in a ventromedial direction 10 to 20 cm lateral to the midline at a point approximately midway between the tuber coxae and the tail head. Pressure should be increased gradually until the horse responds by lifting the lumbar spine, flexing the lumbosacral joint, and bending the haunches away from the pressure (toward the therapist). The movements should occur smoothly and slowly, not in a fast, jerky fashion. This exercise is performed to the left and right sides.

Combined Techniques for Thoracic, Lumbar, and Lumbosacral Lifting

Thoracic lifting can be combined with lumbar and lumbosacral lifting to raise and round the length of the back. Pressure is applied first to the vertebral spines on the dorsal midline or in the intermuscular groove to lift the lumbar and lumbosacral regions, and then pressure is applied to the ventral midline to lift the thoracic region. In small horses, one person can perform the combined stimulations; but large horses may need 2 people.

BALANCING EXERCISES

When the horse is standing still, balance is maintained by keeping the center of mass (COM) within the boundaries of the horizontal base of support.[40] The postural control system responds to perturbations by stimulating muscular activity that adjusts the ground reaction forces to maintain postural balance.[41] When the horse is in motion, it does not need to maintain its COM above the base of support defined by the grounded limbs. Instead, dynamic balance relies on a combination of momentum that keeps the body moving forward as gravity pulls the horse downward until the next limbs contact the ground to support the body and propel it forward.

Perturbations of the standing horse's balance stimulate responses directed toward maintaining the COM within the boundaries of the base of support by adjusting the tension in the extrinsic limb muscles and other core muscles. By perturbing the horse's balance in different directions, it is possible to recruit various components of the core musculature on both sides of the body. Repetition of the exercises leads to improvements in balance and stability. When the horse's COM is shifted caudally, the muscles of the thoracic sling are engaged. If the haunches are pushed laterally, the pelvic stabilizer muscles are recruited. The effects of balancing exercises have not yet been studied experimentally, though there are anecdotal reports of their effects in improving movements, such as canter pirouettes, that require extreme balance and coordination.

Backward Weight Shift

The therapist faces the horse's shoulder with the forward hand placed over the sternum and manubrium and the thumb on the manubrium. Gentle pressure is applied to the manubrium until the horse rocks back slightly. The horse displaces the COM toward the haunches by contracting the thoracic sling muscles, sublumbar muscles, middle gluteal, m tensor fasciae latae, and m biceps femoris. If the therapist's free hand is placed just behind the withers, it is possible to feel the rocking motion as the horse's weight shifts caudally. When pressure is removed, the trunk is seen and felt to move forward. In dogs, it has been shown electromyographically that pushing forward against a caudally directed force increases activity in m multifidi.

Tail Pull

Pulling the tail laterally activates the pelvic stabilizer muscles, primarily biceps femoris, to maintain the horse's balance. The therapist faces the horse's haunches and gently pulls the tail to one side. The horse resists falling sideways by activating the muscles around the hip and stifle and may lean away from the therapist. The goal is not to pull the horse off balance, but simply to stimulate resistance in the pelvic stabilizer muscles. The muscles that are activated in the tail pull are those that prevent excessive motion or laxity during transmission of propulsive forces through the stifle and hip joints. As the muscles get stronger, the amount of force can be gradually increased and the tail pull can be used when the horse is walking.

Destabilizing with a Leg Raised

The therapist picks up a forelimb and raises it to a height that is comfortable for the horse. Sufficient pressure is then applied to the sternum or point of the shoulder to rock the horse's weight back and/or sideways but not enough to cause the horse to stagger sideways. The position is held for 5 seconds, and then the pressure is released. The applied force alternates between pushing straight back toward the ipsilateral hind limb and pushing diagonally back toward the opposite hind limb. The pelvic stabilizer muscles control the weight shift and lateral balance assisted by the thoracic sling muscles, primarily serratus ventralis, on the grounded side.

Combination Exercises

The backward weight shift, the tail pull, and the hind limb destabilizing exercises can be combined with lumbosacral rounding. A second person is needed to apply pressure to the vertebral spines in front of the tail head or in the intermuscular groove.

EXERCISE AT DIFFERENT GAITS AND SPEEDS

The function of the core musculature varies with gait and speed. During walking, m longissimus and m iliocostalis contribute to bending the thoracolumbar spine laterally as the hind limb is protracted and approaches the grounded ipsilateral forelimb.[10,12] As a result, the spine bends away from the protracting hind limb, allowing it to step further forward. Rectus abdominis does not show phasic activity at walk.[42]

During locomotion, most of the movements of the back are driven passively by gravitational, inertial, and ground reaction forces and the epaxial muscles play an important role in controlling or limiting the amount of motion. When trotting and galloping, muscle recruitment increases to provide spinal stability that controls the bouncing motion associated with the suspension phases. During trotting, the epaxial muscles are activated in late stance to limit spinal flexion and the abdominal muscles are activated in early to midstance to limit spinal extension. Thus, both muscles act eccentrically to provide sagittal plane stabilization.[10,12,38,42,43] Activity of m longissimus dorsi is somewhat synchronous on the left and right sides but with greater activity on the side ipsilateral to the hind limb that is retracting and generating propulsive forces.[10,12] At faster trotting speeds, m longissimus dorsi and m rectus abdominis are activated earlier in the stride cycle and with greater intensity, which results in greater spinal stiffness at faster speeds.[37] An increase in trotting speed is also associated with increased activity in the external abdominal oblique muscle[18] and earlier activation of m splenius,[37] which resists downward motion of the neck and increases its rigidity.

At the canter and gallop, thoracolumbar flexion and extension make a significant contribution to stride length. In dogs, the epaxial muscles actively extend the back.[4] In horses, m longissimus is active bilaterally through most of the hind limb swing phases; this has been suggested to maintain hind limb elevation as the hindquarters are protracted.[42] Epaxial muscle activation occurs sequentially in a cranial-to-caudal direction, which resembles the wave patterns generated in more primitive quadrupedal species. The m rectus abdominis is active reciprocally with m longissimus with activity on the side of the trailing hind limb preceding that on the side of the leading hind limb.[42] Trunk stability is particularly important at high speed to provide a stable platform for rapid limb oscillations.[44]

Because the activation and coordination patterns of the core musculature vary between gaits, it is beneficial to use different gaits to stimulate the neuromotor control system to produce diverse and varied patterns of muscle recruitment and coordination. Transitions between gaits involve changing the limb coordination pattern and are regarded as a stimulus to improve neuromotor control. In general, gaits with a suspension phase require higher levels of muscular activity to stabilize the spine, so rehabilitation should start with walking and then progress to trot and canter. The maximal force exerted on the horse's back increases proportionally to the rider's weight and is approximately equal to the rider's weight at walk, double the rider's weight at trot, and almost 3 times the rider's weight at canter.[45] Riding style affects the force pattern. At trot, for example, maximal force is highest in sitting trot with 2 equal maxima in each stride. By comparison, in rising trot, maximal force is slightly lower on the sitting diagonal and markedly lower on the standing diagonal compared with sitting trot.[46] When riding in a light (2-point) seat, the rider stands in the stirrups allowing the hip, knee, and ankle to flex and absorb the vertical motion of the horse, which smoothes the loading pattern so maximal forces are decreased. This effect is particularly apparent in the gallop in which the crouched seat adopted by the jockey actually reduces energy expenditure by the horse.[47] Therefore, in horses that are rehabilitating from a back injury, the initial exercise should be done without a rider. The weight on the back can be increased gradually starting with a weighted saddle pad and progressing to heavier weights then a lightweight rider. When riding in trot and canter, the use of a light seat will decrease the peak load on the horse's back.

Rehabilitative exercise should initially be performed at walk with weekly increases in the walking speed or duration. Walking exercise initiates the conditioning and strengthening of m longissimus. The introduction of trotting significantly increases the activation of the epaxial muscles and recruits m rectus abdominis for sagittal plane stability. When trotting is introduced, it is performed initially for short periods separated by walk breaks and with a weekly increment in trotting duration. An increase in trotting speed provides a further stimulus to muscular activation. An effective way to increase speed is to use speed play.[48] This play involves a gradual acceleration with the faster speed being maintained over a short distance followed by a gradual deceleration to the original speed. Progressive loading is accomplished by increasing the duration or speed of the faster bursts or by performing the transitions more abruptly. Muscle activity increases further when canter or gallop are introduced, and the asymmetrical nature of these gaits challenges the horse's neuromotor control. In contrast to the symmetric gaits, the hypaxial and epaxial muscles may contribute to flexion and extension of the spine, especially the lumbosacral joint. Progressive loading can be accomplished as described for the trot.

EXERCISE ON CIRCLES

Circular locomotion differs from straight locomotion in that it requires a turning or centripetal force acting toward the center of the circle, which accelerates the body in the direction of the turn. The easiest way for the horse to generate a turning force is to lean into the circle.[49,50] Horses trotting slowly (2.3 m/s) around a 6-m diameter circle lean inward by an average of 14.8°.[49] By leaning inwards, the force vector is more closely aligned with the central axis of the limb, thereby reducing tension in the soft tissues on the medial and lateral aspects of the joints, such as the collateral ligaments. However, the limbs on the inside of the turn are oriented at a more acute angle to the ground than the limbs on the outside.[50]

Sport horses are trained to maintain a vertical orientation of the limbs and body when turning. In order to achieve this, the horse uses the abductor and adductor muscles to generate turning forces; working on circles will strengthen these muscle groups. Horses are also trained to bend the spine to match, as closely as possible, the circumference of the circle. The epaxial and oblique abdominal muscles on the inside contract to bend the horse's back in the direction of turning. It requires considerable muscular strength to bend the horse's back because the equine spine is stiffer in lateral bending than in flexion-extension.[51]

Turning and circling exercises can be performed in hand, on long lines, on the lunge, or under a rider. The magnitude of the required turning force increases as the turn radius decreases and as locomotor speed increases, so the training begins on large circles at slow speed. The horse is encouraged to maintain a vertical position, to bend along the circle line, and to perform symmetrically on the left and right reins. The progression involves decreasing the circle size, and the use of a spiral pattern is particularly beneficial. Starting on a large (20 m) circle, the size is gradually reduced by following a spiral path to the smallest diameter on which the horse can comfortably maintain the bend. This circle is maintained for one or 2 revolutions, then the circle size is gradually increased again. As the circle size changes, the horse must coordinate concentric activity in the m longissimus and the oblique abdominal muscles on the inside of the turn with controlled eccentric activity of the contralateral muscles to allow lateral bending and yielding through the ribcage. Over time, improvements in strength and coordination allow the horse to perform correctly on smaller circles. A further progression is to increase the speed, especially at trot, on a large (20–30 m) circle.

Lateral exercises, such as shoulder in, haunches in, or half pass, require the horse to bend the body and cross the forelimbs, the hind limbs, or both during locomotion. These movements activate and strengthen m longissimus dorsi, the abdominal oblique muscles, the abductors, and the adductors.

GRADIENTS

Working the horse on a gradient makes use of the effects of gravity to selectively load the hind limbs on an incline or the forelimbs on a decline. Specifically, walking uphill increases the activation of m longissimus dorsi.[12] Trotting on an incline is associated with increased activity of m longissimus.[37] Studies in dogs have additionally shown that trotting uphill activates m multifidi as well as m longissimus, especially in the lumbar region, whereas activity in both muscles decreases when trotting downhill.[4] The oblique abdominal muscles are recruited to provide sagittal plane stabilization against shearing forces imposed on the axial skeleton by the action of the hind limb retractor muscles on an incline and the hind limb protractor muscles on a decline.[7] When trotting uphill, the large propulsive forces and the accompanying shear forces are controlled by increased activity in the internal abdominal oblique muscles. When going downhill, the hind limb protractor muscles provide a braking effect and the accompanying shear forces are controlled by increased activity in the external abdominal oblique muscles. Although similar studies have not been published in horses, the underlying mechanical principles suggest that the effect will be the same and that exercise on gradients can be used to recruit and strengthen the oblique abdominal muscles. Trotting at medium to fast speeds on a moderate uphill slope is particularly effective for strengthening the epaxial and abdominal muscles.[37,52]

As with other types of exercise, gradients should be incorporated gradually into the exercise routine starting with a small number of repetitions on a gentle slope and incrementally increasing the work by performing a larger number of repetitions or by including steeper gradients. Cantering up gradual gradients is an excellent method of cardiovascular conditioning, whereas steeper uphill gradients strengthen the propulsive muscles in the hindquarters. Because the effects of gravity increase forelimb concussion when traveling downhill, it is recommended that horses descend at walk on anything more than a gradual slope.

The effect of gravitational loading of the forelimbs on a downhill slope is thought to strengthen the extrinsic musculature of the thoracic girdle, specifically m serratus ventralis. The horse must maintain good posture with the forehand and withers elevated (**Fig. 9**). From the rider's perspective, this implies that the horse is not leaning on the bit and each forelimb is loaded in a slow controlled manner. The inclusion of frequent halts, and even some steps of rein back are beneficial. Although not yet confirmed

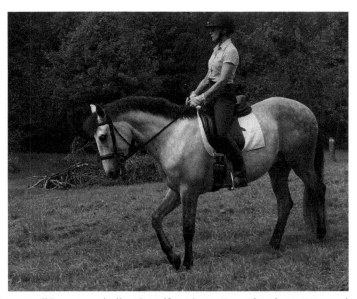

Fig. 9. Horse walking on a decline in self-carriage. Note the short steps and elevation through the withers. (*From* Stubbs NC, Clayton HM. Activate your horse's core. Mason (MI): Sport Horse Publications; 2008; with permission.)

experimentally, anecdotal reports suggest that slow, controlled downhill exercise improves the horse's posture and self-carriage.

JUMPING

In the context of core training, jumping can be likened to uphill locomotion during the take off and to downhill locomotion during the landing. However, at take off, the 2 hind limbs push off fairly symmetrically in terms of their placement relative to the fence and the timing of the propulsive effort, so the force vector is closely aligned with the median plane of the body. The pelvic stabilizing muscles should be engaged to maintain alignment in the frontal plane and facilitate force transmission through the stifle, hip, and pelvis. During the aerial phase, the horse bascules, which involves rounding the back in the absence of ground reaction forces. At landing, the forelimbs are separated temporally and spatially; the trailing forelimb is loaded first followed by the leading forelimb, and the large landing forces create a torque around the ribcage. These forces, which increase with the height of the fence, are likely to stimulate increased activity in the forelimb extrinsic musculature that is recruited to control the descent and rotation of the trunk. Jumping should only be used as a core training exercise in horses that jump in good form with a rounded bascule so that the appropriate muscles are being trained.

POLES

Stepping over poles on the ground or raised above the ground is a different type of exercise than jumping. A jumping horse is airborne while negotiating the fence; but when trotting over poles, one diagonal pair of limbs remains weight-bearing while the other diagonal pair is raised clear of the poles.[53] Therefore, trotting over poles does not involve an exaggerated suspension phase and does not require an increase in propulsive ground reaction forces.[54]

The effort of raising the swing limbs clear of the poles perturbs the horse's balance and obligates the stance limbs to provide balance and stability. The forelimbs show a small but significant increase in peak braking force and a larger, significant increase in braking impulse when trotting over poles, which implies recruitment of the extensor musculature, likely including the thoracic sling muscles, such as m serratus ventralis. The forelimbs also show a change from a net medially directed transverse impulse to a net laterally directed impulse, which implies activity of the adductors, such as the pectoral muscles, to maintain the vertical alignment of the forelimbs.[54] Thus, trotting over poles benefits core training by strengthening the extrinsic forelimb musculature (extensors and adductors) and may also recruit the core stabilizing musculature.

UNSTABLE FOOTING

Human physical therapists often make use of an unstable surface, such as a Swiss ball or BOSU Balance Trainer, to challenge the motor control system. Increased activity has been demonstrated in the core mobilizing musculature when performing core training exercises on an unstable surface.[55] More specifically, when abdominal curl-up exercises are performed on an unstable surface muscle activity increases and there are changes in the abdominal muscle coactivation patterns that stabilize the spine and the whole body, which suggests greater demands on the motor control system.[56] It is not unreasonable to speculate that there might be value for horses to perform dynamic mobilization and core training exercises on an unstable surface to

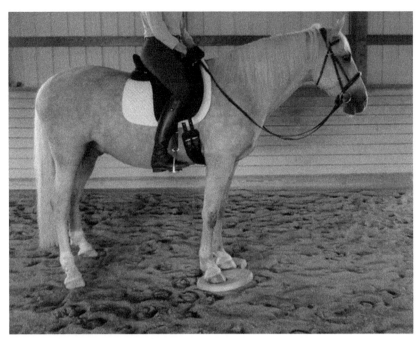

Fig. 10. Horse standing on Sure Foot cushions. (*Courtesy of* Sure Foot Equine Stability Program, Washington, VA; with permission.)

provide a further challenge for horses that are already familiar with performing core training exercises on stable footing.

A selection of durable, low-profile balance cushions and pads suitable for this purpose are available for horses (Sure Foot, Equine Stability Program, Murdoch Method, Washington, VA). The Sure Foot cushions provide a safe and apparently comfortable experience for the horse, with most horses standing willingly and relaxing as they become accustomed to the cushions (**Fig. 10**). The cushions can be placed under one or more feet; different combinations of feet, for example, contralateral, ipsilateral, or diagonal pairs, can be placed on the cushions. After the horse is comfortable standing on the unstable surface, a progression of the degree of difficulty is to raise one limb and apply a small perturbation to the horse's body. A further progression is to perform DMEs while standing on the cushions. Initially the chin is moved through a small distance with a gradual increase as the horse's stability improves.

Walking over an unstable surface, such as a mattress or soft rubber pad, can also be used to challenge the horse's core stability and motor control. The therapist must ensure that the surface is safe and not slippery. Unstable surfaces are useful for recruiting the core muscles in all horses and especially for rehabilitating horses with neurologic problems that have reached an appropriate stage of recovery.

REFERENCES

1. Townsend HGG, Leach DH. Relationship between intervertebral joint morphology and mobility in the equine thoracolumbar spine. Equine Vet J 1984;15:461–5.
2. Slijper EJ. Comparative biologic-anatomical investigations on the vertebral column and spinal musculature of mammals. Proc K Ned Acad Wetensch 1946; 42:1–128.

3. Stubbs NC, Hodges PW, Jeffcott LB, et al. Functional anatomy of the caudal thoracolumbar and lumbosacral spine in the horse. Equine Vet J 2006;(Suppl 36): 393–9.
4. Schilling N, Carrier DR. Function of the epaxial muscles in walking, trotting and galloping dogs: implications for the evolution of epaxial muscle function in tetrapods. J Exp Biol 2010;213:1490–502.
5. Hodges J, Richardson C. Feed forward contraction of transverse abdominis is not influenced by the direction of an arm movement. Exp Brain Res 1997;114: 362–70.
6. Hall LW, Aziz HA, Groenendyk J, et al. Electromyography of some respiratory muscles in the horse. Res Vet Sci 1991;50:328–33.
7. Fife MM, Bailey CL, Lee DV, et al. Function of the oblique hypaxial muscles in trotting dogs. J Exp Biol 1991;204:2371–81.
8. Hyytiäinen HK, Mykkänen AK, Hielm-Björkman AK, et al. Muscle fibre type distribution of the thoracolumbar and hindlimb regions of horses: relating fibre type and functional role. Acta Vet Scand 2014;56:8. Available at: http://www.actavetscand.com/content/56/1/8.
9. Bogduk M, Twomey L. The lumbar muscles and their fasci. In: Bogduk N, Twomey L, editors. Clinical anatomy of the lumbar spine. London: Churchill Livingston; 1987. p. 75–116.
10. Licka T, Frey A, Peham C. Electromyographic activity of the longissimus dorsi muscles in horses when walking on a treadmill. Vet J 2009;180:71–6.
11. Wakeling JM, Barnett K, Price S, et al. Effects of manipulative therapy on the longissimus dorsi in the equine back. Equine Compar Exerc Physiol 2006;3: 153–60.
12. Wakeling JM, Ritruechaia P, Dalton S, et al. Segmental variation in the activity and function of the equine longissimus dorsi muscle during walk and trot. Compar Exerc Physiol 2007;4:95–103.
13. McGowan CM, Hodges PW, Jeffcott LB. Epaxial musculature and its relationship with back pain in the horse. In: RIRDC horse projects completed in 2006-07 and horse research in progress as at June 2007. Barton, ACT, Australia: Rural Industries Research and Development Corporation; 2007. p. 37.
14. Holm KR, Wennerstrand J, Lagerquist U, et al. Effect of local analgesia on movement of the equine back. Equine Vet J 2006;38:65–9.
15. Stubbs NC, Riggs CM, Clayton HM, et al. Spinal pathology and epaxial muscle ultrasonography in thoroughbred racehorses. Equine Vet J 2010;42(Suppl 38): 654–61.
16. Hoy D, Brooks P, Blyth F, et al. The epidemiology of low back pain. Best Pract Res Clin Rheum 2010;24:769–81.
17. Jeffcott LB. Disorders of the thoracolumbar spine of the horse. Equine Vet 1980; 12:197–210.
18. Townsend HGG, Leach DH, Doige CE, et al. Relationship between spinal biomechanics and pathological changes in the equine thoracolumbar spine. Equine Vet J 1986;18:107–12.
19. Haussler KK, Stover SM, Willits NH. Pathologic changes in the lumbosacral vertebrae and pelvis in Thoroughbred racehorses. Am J Vet Res 1999;60:143–53.
20. de Oliveira K, Soutello RVG, da Fonseca R, et al. Gymnastic training and dynamic mobilization exercises improve stride quality and epaxial muscle size in therapy horses. J Equine Vet Sci 2015;35:888–93.
21. Tabor G. The effect of dynamic mobilisation exercises on the equine multifidus muscle and thoracic profile [MS thesis]. Plymouth, UK: Plymouth University; 2015.

22. Stubbs NC, Kaiser LJ, Hauptman J, et al. Dynamic mobilization exercises increase cross sectional area of musculus multifidus. Equine Vet J 2011;43: 522–9.

23. Hodges P, Holm AK, Hansson T, et al. Rapid atrophy of the lumbar multifidus follows experimental disc or nerve root injury. Spine 2006;31:2926–33.

24. Danneels LA, Vanderstraeten GG, Cambier DC, et al. Effects of three different training modalities on the cross sectional area of the lumbar multifidus muscle in patients with chronic low back pain. Br J Sports Med 2001;35:186–91.

25. Hides J, Richardson C, Jull G. Multifidus muscle recovery is not automatic after resolution of acute, first episode low back pain. Spine 1996;21:2763–9.

26. Hides J, Gilmore C, Stanton W, et al. Multifidus size and symmetry among chronic LBP and healthy asymptomatic subjects. Man Ther 2008;13:43–9.

27. Kavcic N, Grenier S, McGill SM. Determining the stabilizing role of individual torso muscles during rehabilitation exercises. Spine 2004;29:1254–65.

28. Hides JA, Jull GA, Richardson CA. Long-term effects of specific stabilizing exercises for first-episode low back pain. Spine 2001;26:E243–8.

29. Ranner W, Gerhards H, Klee W. Diagnostic validity of palpation in horses with back problems. Berl Munch Tierarztl Wochenschr 2002;11:420–4.

30. Munroe GA. The investigation of back pathology: the clinical examination. In: Henson MD, editor. Equine back pathology: diagnosis and treatment. Blackwell publishing; 2009. p. 63–73.

31. Payne RC, Veenman P, Wilson AM. The role of the extrinsic thoracic limb muscles in equine locomotion. J Anat 2004;205:479–90.

32. De Cocq P, van Weeren PR, Back W. Effects of girth, saddle and weight on movements of the horse. Equine Vet J 2004;36:758–63.

33. Jull GA, Richardson CA. Motor control problems in patients with spinal pain: a new direction for therapeutic exercise. J Manipulative Physiol Ther 2002;23: 115–7.

34. Stubbs NC, Clayton HM. Part 1: mobilization exercises. In: Activate your horse's core. Mason (MI): Sport Horse Publications; p. 10–9.

35. Clayton HM, Kaiser LJ, Lavagnino M, et al. Dynamic mobilizations in cervical flexion: effects on intervertebral angulations. Equine Vet J 2010;42(Suppl 38): 688–94.

36. Clayton HM, Kaiser LJ, Lavagnino M, et al. Intervertebral angulations in dynamic mobilizations performed in cervical lateral bending. Am J Vet Res 2012;73: 1153–9.

37. Robert C, Valette JP, Denoix JM. The effects of treadmill inclination and speed on the activity of three trunk muscles in the trotting horse. Equine Vet J 2001;33: 466–72.

38. Stubbs NC, Clayton HM. Core strengthening exercises. In: Activate your horse's core. Mason (MI): Sport Horse Publications; p. 20–4.

39. Peham C, Frey A, Licka T, et al. Evaluation of the EMG activity of the long back muscle during induced back movements in stance. Equine Vet 2001;(Suppl 33):165–8.

40. Røgind H, Lykkegaard JJ, Bliddal H, et al. Postural sway in normal subjects aged 20–70 years. Clin Physiol Funct Imaging 2003;23:171–6.

41. Pavol MJ. Detecting and understanding differences in postural sway: focus on "a new interpretation of spontaneous sway measures based on a simple model of human postural control". J Neurophysiol 2005;93:20–1.

42. Tokuriki M, Otsuki R, Kai M, et al. Electromyographic activity of trunk muscles during locomotion on a treadmill. J Equine Vet Sci 1997;17:468.

43. Robert C, Valette JP, Denoix JM. Surface electromyography analysis of the normal horse locomotion: a preliminary report. In: Proceedings, conference on equine sports medicine and science. The Netherlands: Wageningen Pers; 1998. p. 80–5.

44. Rooney JR. The horse's back: biomechanics and lameness. Equine Pract 1982;4: 17–27.

45. Fruehwirth B, Peham C, Scheidl M, et al. Evaluation of pressure distribution under an English saddle at walk, trot and canter. Equine Vet J 2004;36:754–7.

46. de Cocq P, Duncker AM, Clayton HM, et al. Vertical forces on the horse's back in sitting and rising trot. J Biomech 2010;43:327–631.

47. Pfau T, Spence A, Starke S, et al. Modern riding style improves horse racing times. Science 2009;325:289.

48. Clayton HM. Cardiovascular conditioning. In: Conditioning sport horses. Mason (MI): Sport Horse Publications; 1991. p. 101–2.

49. Clayton HM, Sha DH. Body centre of mass movement in horses travelling on a circular path. Equine Vet J Suppl 2006;36:462–7.

50. Hobbs SJ, Licka T, Polman R. The difference in kinematics of horses walking, trotting and cantering on a flat and banked 10 m circle. Equine Vet J 2011;43: 686–94.

51. Peham C, Schobesberger H. Influence of the load of a rider or of a region with increased stiffness on the equine back: a modeling study. Equine Vet J 2004; 36:703–5.

52. Robert C, Valette JP, Pourcelot P, et al. Effects of trotting speed on muscle activity and kinematics in saddlehorses. Equine Vet J 2002;(Suppl 34):295–301.

53. Brown S, Stubbs N, Kaiser L, et al. Swing phase kinematics of horses trotting over poles. Equine Vet J 2015;47:107–12.

54. Clayton HM, Brown S, Lavagnino M, et al. Stance phase kinematics and ground reaction forces of horses trotting over poles. Equine Vet J 2015;47:113–8.

55. Imai A, Kaneoka K, Okubo Y, et al. Trunk muscle activity during lumbar stabilization exercises on both a stable and unstable surface. J Orthop Sports Phys Ther 2010;40:369–75.

56. Vera-Garcia FJ, Grenier SG, McGill SM. Abdominal muscle response during curl-ups on both stable and labile surfaces. Phys Ther 2000;80:564–9.

Acupuncture and Equine Rehabilitation

Sarah le Jeune, DVM[a],*, Kimberly Henneman, DVM[b], Kevin May, DVM[c]

KEYWORDS

- Acupuncture • Integrative medicine • Rehabilitation

KEY POINTS

- Acupuncture is one of the most common veterinary integrative medicine modalities.
- Acupuncture can greatly contribute to a rehabilitation protocol by promoting analgesia, tissue healing, and muscle strength.
- Acupuncture is safe, has minimal detrimental side effects, and is well tolerated by most horses.

INTRODUCTION

Recent advances in sport horse medicine and rehabilitation have made it possible for equine athletes to reach new levels of excellence. Client demand for superior diagnostics and innovative treatment strategies requires equine practitioners to be more informed than ever before. In addition to Western advances in sport horse medicine, acupuncture for the equine athlete has become increasingly recognized as an effective and valuable tool to treat musculoskeletal conditions associated with the demands of intensive physical conditioning and performance and to aid in rehabilitating musculoskeletal injuries.

A 2008 survey conducted by the American Association of Equine Practitioners identified that 20% of equine practitioner respondents perform some form of integrative medicine treatment modality themselves (most commonly acupuncture and chiropractic) and, of those who do not, 80% refer cases specifically for complementary medicine to veterinarians who have this expertise. Currently most of the veterinary institutions in North America offer some form of integrative medicine, primarily acupuncture and chiropractic, in their clinical services and veterinary curriculum.

The authors have nothing to disclose.
[a] Department of Surgical and Radiological Sciences, University of California, Davis, CA 95616, USA; [b] Animal Health Options, Park City, UT 84098, USA; [c] Department of Equine, El Cajon Valley Veterinary Hospital, 560 North Johnson Avenue, El Cajon, CA 92020, USA
* Corresponding author.
E-mail address: sslejeune@ucdavis.edu

Vet Clin Equine 32 (2016) 73–85
http://dx.doi.org/10.1016/j.cveq.2015.12.004
0749-0739/16/$ – see front matter © 2016 Elsevier Inc. All rights reserved.
vetequine.theclinics.com

Horse owners are attracted to acupuncture because it is safe, has minimal detrimental side effects, and is well tolerated by most horses. Horses experiencing performance issues associated with musculoskeletal pain, and who must comply with prohibited substance policies mandated by show associations, can benefit showside from acupuncture and/or chiropractic treatments. This occurs at most elite competitions in compliance with the Fédération Equèstre Internationale (FEI) Sports.

Acupuncture is often sought directly by horse owners, sometimes without the involvement of their primary veterinarian, leading to a disconnection between this modality and traditional veterinary medicine. This has caused the creation of a rift between conventional medicine and integrative medicine, which is to the detriment of the horse: both practices can be mutually beneficial and rich in information that can optimize a patient's treatment response.

The goals of veterinary physical rehabilitation are to reduce pain; facilitate tissue healing; restore muscle strength, endurance, and proprioception; and restore the animal to its prior level of activity while preventing further injury. Acupuncture can greatly contribute to a rehabilitation protocol by promoting analgesia, tissue healing, and muscle strength.

Lameness is commonly encountered during a rehabilitation program and acupuncture can be used not only in the treatment but also in the detection of lameness in horses. Most horse owners cannot adequately detect lameness until it is severe, that is, present at the walk or trot. Recently, a prospective study was conducted to answer the question of whether palpation or scanning for reactive acupuncture points (acupoints) could be useful in screening for lameness in performance horses.[1] The study population consisted of 102 performance horses (jumpers, dressage horses, and Western performance horses) evenly distributed into lame and sound groups. These horses first underwent an acupuncture scan and then a routine lameness examination. The results of this study show that 78% (40/51) of sound horses were negative during the acupuncture scan (did not have a painful response at any of the acupuncture points palpated), whereas, only 18% (9/51) of lame horses were negative during the acupuncture scan ($P<.001$), indicating that acupuncture scanning has a sensitivity of 82.4% in detecting lameness and a specificity of 78.4%. This suggests that horses that have a positive acupuncture scan should undergo a lameness examination to identify the presence and source of their lameness. The information provided by the acupuncture scan could also be useful while following a horse during rehabilitation of a musculoskeletal injury.

Acupuncture can certainly be used to help relieve pain in many musculoskeletal conditions, but it is critical that the primary cause also be addressed with traditional methods. Back pain is common in riding horses and can be difficult to diagnose and treat with conventional methods. Back pain is a good example of a term that encompasses a wide variety of conditions, with just as many causes. Horses experiencing chronic pain typically have a loss of performance and can also exhibit withdrawn social behavior and possibly experience a decreased appetite with subsequent decreased nutritional intake. This is due to the effect of chronic pain on the emotional centers of the limbic system, which motivates the individual to withdraw from damaging situations, to protect a damaged body part while it heals, and to avoid similar experiences in the future.[2–5]

The human model of spinal rehabilitation includes a multidisciplinary approach in the management of back problems. Advances in the treatment of equine back pain incorporate some of the same philosophies. The difficulty lies in identifying the exact cause of back pain, because it is often multifactorial. Back pain is commonly associated with lameness and it is critical to identify whether a horse is suffering from primary back pain or if the back pain is secondary to limb lameness. Horses with back pain should, therefore, undergo a full lameness examination, potentially with limb blocks to rule out lower limb lameness. In addition, factors, such as saddle fit, tack fit, dental status, shoeing, conditioning program, and rider ability, should be assessed when dealing with back pain cases. Several studies report that acupuncture is effective in treating back pain in horses.[6,7] In the author's (SLJ) experience, it takes at least 3 consecutive (weekly) treatments to obtain a long-lasting clinical resolution of back pain and these horses can then benefit from regular (monthly) acupuncture treatments. The duration and quality of the therapeutic effect may be improved by incorporating chiropractic treatments in addition to acupuncture, but clinical studies are needed to confirm this clinical impression.

HISTORY OF ACUPUNCTURE

Acupuncture has been a part of Traditional Chinese Veterinary Medicine (TCVM) for centuries. Ma Shihuang was considered the first man to treat animal diseases with acupuncture and herbal medicine (2696 BCE to 2598 BCE).[8] Sun Yang, also known as Bo Le (659 BCE–621 BCE), wrote what is considered the first veterinary acupuncture text, *Bo Le's Canon of Veterinary Acupuncture*.[8,9] Since that time, veterinary acupuncture has continued to evolve and is an integral part of TCVM. In more recent times, this form of healing has branched out to the rest of the world and is becoming integrated into the health care of animal patients. Starting in the early 1970s, the United States saw the formation of the International Veterinary Acupuncture Society, which started offering training courses in veterinary acupuncture to licensed veterinarians. By 2000, there were additional educational opportunities in veterinary acupuncture available from The Chi Institute and One Health Scientific Integrative Medicine. Today, acupuncture is included as an integral part of veterinary medicine programs in both academic institutions and private clinics around the world.[10]

MECHANISMS OF ACTION
Acupoints

Acupoints are focal areas where needles are routinely inserted through the skin (or pressure exerted topically for acupressure) to exert a physiologic effect. Although debate still exists as to what an acupoint is structurally, these areas have been shown to possess unique biophysical characteristics functionally and physiologically. Changes in electric, acoustic, thermal, optical, magnetic, isotopic, and myoelectric responses of acupoints have been shown to differ from surrounding, nonacupoint tissue.[11]

There are 2 types of acupuncture points that are available for therapeutic use in injury rehabilitation: classical Asian meridian or channel points (the organ and extraordinary meridians) and nonmeridian points. Nonmeridian points are often called *ashi* (ā shì xué) points and are often considered the equivalent of myofascial trigger points. These points are identified by their reactivity and sensitivity to touch.[12] Although classic meridian points are predictably found in the same anatomic locations, ashi points are often variable (but not necessarily so), unpredictable, and appear relative to individual symptoms.[13]

Even fixed location meridian points are still actively dynamic in response to pathology, changing in sensitivity, size, and reactivity. Reactivity is categorized as latent (normal), passive (pain only on stimulation), or active (constant pain)[13]; 70% of classical acupuncture points can also be classified as trigger points due to their association with skeletal muscles.[14] Reactivity of an acupuncture point develops when local or systemic homeostasis is disturbed; passive and active points can be recognized by the presence of pain, higher surface temperature, and significantly increased electrical conductivity. Ashi points tend to be unilateral, in contrast to reactive points associated with homeostatic or global dysfunction, which tend to be symmetric.

Acupoints have been demonstrated to have close relationships to nerves. Rarely, however, does needling of a classical meridian or extrameridian point actually involve penetrating a major nerve trunk with a needle (except perhaps by accident); if it did, it is doubtful that most animals would allow a veterinary acupuncturist to ever insert a needle again. Acupoints are perhaps more closely associated with fascia than they are with nerves. These connective tissue, fascial planes are instrumental in the creation of the *de qi*, or tissue grasp sensation, as well as in the mechanical signaling to surrounding tissue (including nerves) that may initiate the acupuncture response (**Fig. 1**). Recent research in humans has generated computer simulations of fascia-rich areas and is correlating them closely to classical acupuncture meridians and collaterals as well as correlating common classical acupuncture points with fascial muscle planes.[15,16] It has also been proposed that the stimulation of differentiation of stored fascial stem cells (mesenchymal) may be one of the mechanisms by which traditional Asian therapies work.[17]

The following nerve structures are closely associated with acupoints (but do not make up the acupoint structure itself)[18]:

- Cutaneous or muscular nerve trunks
- Superficial nerves
- Areas where nerve trunks penetrate through fascia
- Area where nerve trunks emerge from bone foramina
- Neuromuscular attachments
- Neurovascular bundles

Neurologic Mechanisms of Acupuncture Action

The neurophysiologic mechanisms of acupuncture, especially for the management of both acute and chronic pain, are well documented. There is no shortage of

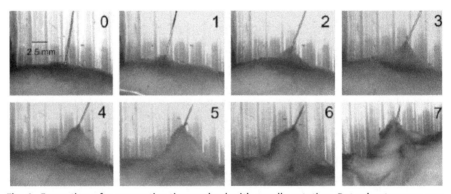

Fig. 1. Formation of a connective tissue whorl with needle rotation. Rat subcutaneous connective tissue was dissected and placed in physiologic buffer under a dissecting microscope. An acupuncture needle was inserted through the tissue and progressively rotated. Numbers 0 through 7 indicate numbers of needle revolutions. A visible whorl of connective tissue can be seen with as little as 1 revolution of the needle. (*From* Langevin HM, Yandow JA. Relationship of acupuncture points and meridians to connective tissue planes. Anat Rec 2002;269(6):260; with permission.)

well-designed human and animal studies that evaluate the effects of acupuncture in cases of cerebral ischemia, reperfusion brain injury, opiate and nonopiate (monoamines, serotonin, norepinephrine, and cytokines) pain modulation, hippocampal nitric oxide synthase activity, and expression of numerous mediators of neurologic inflammation.

Acupuncture can produce many effects on neurologic tissue and function. Because the mechanisms of acupuncture for pain are among the most heavily researched aspects, and because pain management is a topic of significant importance to rehabilitation veterinarians, however, the focus of this paragraph is on those processes. Acupuncture analgesic action can be divided into peripheral and central nervous system effects, although both actions occur together. Central nervous system responses can occur at both spinal segmental and supraspinal nonsegmental levels.[19]

Symptomatic (ashi) points are processed segmentally in the spinal cord and supraspinal areas (midbrain, thalamus, pituitary, and brain cortex).[20] Stimulation of more distal, active meridian points that tend to be more a reflection of homeostatic imbalance are mostly processed nonsegmentally in the supraspinal central nervous system. Both mechanisms are closely interrelated and provide redundancy by enhancing the other's descending control mechanisms. These control mechanisms include the secretion of opiates, sympathetic/parasympathetic neurotransmitters, and hormones that modulate pain and affect immune, endocrine, digestive, cardiovascular, and emotional systems. Achieving the maximum and most sustained results, especially in chronic cases, may dictate a careful and balanced selection by veterinary acupuncturists of both symptomatic (ashi) and homeostatic (classical Asian meridian) points. Because the neurologic aspect of acupuncture analgesia is well explained in many articles and books, the fascial mechanism of acupuncture and its implications to rehabilitative veterinarians are reviewed.

Connective Tissue and Fascial Mechanisms

When a needle penetrates the dermis, a host of cascading, local responses is triggered by the tissue (mostly fascia and myofiber) deformation and damage caused by the needle penetration. Not only has issue distortion caused by an acupuncture needle entering tissue been demonstrated[21,22] but also this distortion can vary anisotropically relative to the needle location.[22] When a needle was placed trigger-point style in a muscle belly made up mostly of contractile myofibers, the tissue displacement and strain (deformation) response was transverse across the cross-section of a particular muscle unit; when needling occurred between muscle fibers into the fascial septa, then the tissue deformation response was directed longitudinally along the length of the total unit of myofibers, tendons and fascial tissue.[23] Thus, different signaling results from the varied deformations traveling through fascial planes from the 2 different acupuncture techniques (classical meridian vs trigger point). This in turn results in different responses in muscle fibers (and connected nerve networks) and supportive connective tissues (and contained neurovascular bundles), which may explain the response variations in neurologic signaling and information processing.

The global body fascial system is actually one of the most complex systems of the body. Made of mostly type I collagen fibers and fibroblasts, the fibroblasts control the production of collagen and extracellular matrix (ECM) as well as the opening and closing of fascial water pores. The total body connectivity of more superficial muscle with deeper visceral fascial layers has been demonstrated in the human.[24] Visceral fascia is organized into 4 main layers: muscular fascia surrounding body wall muscles, the fascia of the neurovascular bundles, the fascia surrounding individual organs, and the fascia supporting the pleural and peritoneal linings,[25,26] all of which are highly innervated as well as having direct biomechanical connections to muscular fascia. Both visceral and myofascial layers support and protect critical signaling neurovascular bundles[24]; additionally, the cellular (fibroblast) aspect of the fascia is sensitive to changes in force application to the cell membrane as well as changes in local environmental factors, such as pH, pressure, electricity, water, and chemical compositions— all of which can be altered by acupuncture.[27] Due to the interwoven relationships (called *fascial chains* or *trains*)[28,29] of these various fascial tissues, internal organs are part of a continuous woven body matrix rich in nerves, blood vessels, fibroblasts, mesenchymal stem cells, proteins, water, and electrolytes that reaches from the base of the skull into the pelvic cavity and down the spinal muscles. These same total body myofascial connections have recently been demonstrated in the horse.[30]

When a fine metal filament (acupuncture needle) is used to puncture a spot on the skin that has been identified as a treatment acupoint, a profound and multifaceted response cascades through many cellular and tissue functions. A significant majority of classical acupuncture points are associated with fascial connective tissue planes. When the needle penetrates the skin at the location of a classical acupoint or trigger point, it enters into the loose subdermal and intermuscular connective tissue made of reactive fibroblasts and linked collagen fiber bundles.

As the acupuncturist twists the needle to achieve deqi, or needle grasp, the collagen fibers start to grip and wind around the needle, stretching and straightening, radiating the deformation distal from where the needle is inserted. This stretching of the collagen in the fascial network of connective tissue and water disturbs the nestling fibroblasts into responding immediately through various signaling, which includes the release of ATP and the analgesic, inhibitory neurotransmitter adenosine.[31] The cytoskeleton of the fibroblast also starts the process of transforming into a contractile fibroblast within minutes of being exposed to the environmental mechanical deformations.[16,32,33]

This deformed and transformed contractile myofibroblast regulates the production of the local ECM. It can, therefore, alter fluid flow and tissue rigidity in response to trauma (including that caused by a needle), which in turn can affect the ability of cells to adhere to the ECM as well as to other cells.[27] When local cell contacts are broken by the environmental mechanical deformation, autocrine and paracrine reactions lead to the release of cellular growth factors, kinase cascades (protein synthesis initiator), cytokines, cyclooxygenase-2, and nitric oxide enzymes and peptides. Gene activation also occurs, including those for protein synthesis, gene transcription factors, and even proto-oncogenes.[31,34] Contraction and straightening of grasping collagen fibers from the pulling of a manipulated needle cause progressive mechanical recruitment of additional, more distant fibers, thereby creating a transmitting signal of ECM deformation and additional cell contraction, which in turn affects the organism at many levels, including gene expression, neurologic response, pain, immune function, and local cellular chemical and tissue water regulation.

Fascial physiology and response to deformation can explain a concept that is important for rehabilitation veterinarians to keep in mind—overstimulation of a point. All the fascia in the body is connected to itself, from the loose superficial to the dense investing layer of muscles to the fascicular tubes of tendon, ligament, and neurovascular bundles; it is essentially "an uninterrupted viscoelastic tissue which forms a 3-D collagen matrix" that is "virtually inseparable from all structures of the body and acts to create continuity amongst tissues...".[25] Within this collagen matrix are the transiting neurovascular bundles that serve the body, from brain (the dura and pia maters are also connective tissue fascia) to spine to neuromuscular junction. It has been shown in vitro that when type I collagen gels were biomechanically stressed with computer-rotated needles at a set frequency and number of revolutions, collagen failure was more apt to occur in the collagen that had the greater levels of cross-linking.[21] In vivo, aging leads to increased cross-linking of collagen fibers[35] and decreased collagen content.[36] Cross-linking is associated with decreased tissue flexibility and dynamic response, whereas decreased collagen content is associated with fragility and an inability for the ECM to adhese and hold together through nonfunctional catch bonds. This research information should be considered when dealing with elderly animals or in areas of significant trauma because there is potential to do harm with vigorous acupuncture in older collagen tissue or that containing substantial scarring.

Neurogenic Regeneration

Electroacupuncture for the treatment and rehabilitation of peripheral nerve and spinal cord injuries seems promising. In rat models of spinal cord injury, electroacupuncture contributed to the proliferation of neural stem cells in the injured spinal cord, promoting spinal cord repair.[37] Findings of a recent study using a rat model of brain hypoxia indicate that 15-Hz and 30-Hz electroacupuncture of acupoints ST36 and LI11 can favorably maintain the structural integrity of astrocytes, which play a protective role in cerebral ischemic injury.[38]

For treatment and rehabilitation of peripheral nerve injuries, many acupuncture clinicians focus on the injury site, selecting acupoints exclusively along the injured nerve trunk. It seems, however, that peripheral nerve injury not only affects the actual location of the injury but also can induce neuronal apoptosis at the level of the spinal cord. Neglecting to treat centrally may, therefore, delay the onset of treatment efficacy and rehabilitation, as recently evidenced by a study on the optimal selection of acupoints for the treatment of human patients with peripheral nerve injuries.[39] The results of that study indicate that Governing vessel (GV) acupoints, centrally along the dorsal midline, and local meridian acupoints used simultaneously for electroacupuncture stimulation enhance functional repair after peripheral nerve injury. A good clinical response was obtained after 6 weeks of treatments for 30 minutes, once a day, 5 times per week, in 80% of the patients treated locally and centrally (GV meridian) as opposed to only 38.5% in the peripherally treated group. In addition, in 1 patient with radial nerve paresis, electromyography was performed before, during, and after electroacupuncture. After a single treatment of electroacupuncture at GV acupoints, the patient's motor nerve conduction velocity increased by 23.2%.

Based on clinical and scientific evidence, acupuncture can be used in a rehabilitation protocol to aid in

1. Pain control
2. Edema reduction
3. Muscle spasm reduction
4. Vasodilation
5. Neuronal regeneration
6. Scar tissue reduction

Frequency of treatments and treatment protocols are variable and dependent on the individual acupuncturist and the condition treated. In acute, severe conditions, treatments may be administered daily, particularly if analgesia and neuronal stimulation are the ultimate goals.

THERAPEUTIC POINTS RECOMMENDED FOR SPECIFIC CONDITIONS
Cervical Vertebral Malformation and/or Cervical Pain with or Without Proprioceptive Deficits

- Dorsal and ventral paravertebral points (Jing-Jia-Ji)[40–46]
- Cervical 9 points (Jiu-Wei)

- (Large Intestine) LI 18, LI 16, LI 11, LI 10, LI 4, LI 1
- (Lung) LU 7
- ST 4, ST 9, ST 10, ST 36, ST 45
- GB 20, GB 21, GB 39, GB 44
- BL 10, BL 11, BL 60, BL 62, BL 67
- (Triple Heater) TH 16, TH 15, TH 5, TH 1
- (Small Intestine) SI 16, SI 3, SI 1
- Chou-Jin, GV 20, GV 16, GV 14, Bai-Hui, GV 2, Wei-Gen, Wei-Jian
- Xi-Mai, luo-Ling-Wu, luo-Zhen

Facial Nerve Paresis

- BL 1, BL 10
- ST 2, ST 4, ST 6, ST 7, ST 36
- LI 20, LI 19, LI 18, LI 11, LI 10, LI 4
- GB 1, GB 2, GB 20, GB 21, GB 39, GB 44
- TH 23, TH 21, TH 17
- SI 19
- Fen-Shui, Jia-Cheng-Jiang, Kai-Guan, Bao-Sai, Mian-Shen-Jing
- (Liver) LIV 3
- GV 20, GV 26, GV 27, Fen-Shui
- CV 24

Laryngeal Hemiplegia

- LI 18
- ST 9, ST 4

Suprascapular Nerve Paresis (Sweeney)

- SI 9, SI 13
- GB 21, GB 22, GB 23
- TH 15, TH 14
- LI 16, LI 15
- LU 7
- Cervical 9 points (Jiu-Wei)
- GV points
- Classical acupuncturists may perform pneumopuncture over atrophied area. Traditionally, this is done at the most dorsal point of the atrophied area and then the air is pushed down.

Radial Nerve Paresis

- LI 16, LI 15, LI 11, LI 10, LI 4, LI 1
- SI 9
- LU 5
- Zhou-Shu (Elbow Association Point)
- TH 14, TH 5
- Cervical 9 points (Jiu-Wei)
- GV points

Wither Pain

- LU 11
- (Pericardium) PC 9
- (Heart) HT 9

- BL 11, BL 12, BL 13, BL 25
- Hua-Tuo-Jia-Ji points in caudal lumbar area
- Mishizaka points in caudal lumbar area
- Iliac point
- Bai-Hui

Thoracolumbar Pain

- Bai-Hui
- Yao-Qian, Yao-Zhong, Yao-Hou
- Hua-Tuo-Jia-Ji points, cranial and caudal to problem area (use points in caudal lumbar area first if possible)
- Mishizaka points, cranial and caudal to problem area (use most cranial sensitive points first)
- Ishizaka points, cranial and caudal to problem area (use most cranial sensitive points first)
- GV points, cranial and caudal to problem area but void caudal withers area
- BL points, cranial and caudal problem area. Caution: from BL 12 to BL 17, it may be necessary to use points from the outer (BL 41 to BL 46) versus inner BL channel, to avoid muscle spasms, violent patient objection, and needle breakage.
- BL 67
- LV 13

Caudal Lumbar and/or Pelvic Pain and Stiffness

- Bai-Hui
- Yan-Chi
- GB-DTC
- GB 27, GB 44
- BL 27, BL 40, BL 51, BL 52, BL 54, BL 67
- Shen-Peng, Shen-Shu, and Shen-Jiao
- LIV 13
- Iliac points
- Hua-Tuo-Jia-Ji, Mishizaka and Ishizaka points (in caudal lumbar area)

Sacroiliac Region Pain or Cauda Equina

- Bai-Hui
- GV 1, GV 2
- Wei-Gen
- Wei-Jian
- Shen-Peng, Shen-Shu, and Shen-Jiao
- Hua-Tuo-Jia-Ji, Mishizaka and Ishizaka points (in caudal lumbar area)
- Iliac points
- Sacral point
- BL 27, BL 31 to BL 34, BL 40, BL 67
- (Kidney) KI 27
- Ba-Shan

Intermittent Upward Fixation of the Patella

- (Spleen) SP 9, SP 10
- Shen-Peng, Shen-Shu, and Shen-Jiao
- Any/all ashi points in lumbosacral area

- Bai-Hui
- ST 35 and Medial Xiyan

Thoracic Limb Pain (Including Postoperative on Distal Limb)

- SI 9
- TH 5
- LI 4, LI 10, LI 18
- All Jing-Well (ting) points for involved channels

Rear Limb Pain/Weakness

- All Jing-Well (ting) points for involved channels/meridians
- Bai-Hui
- BL 40, BL 54, BL 60
- ST 36
- GB 34, GB 39

Chronic Debilitating Conditions

- ST 36
- LI 10
- Qi-Hai-Shu
- LI 4
- LIV 3
- SP 6

Appetite Stimulation

- GV 25
- Mi-Jiao-Gan

REFERENCES

1. le Jeune SS, Jones JH. Prospective study on the correlation of positive acupuncture scans and lameness in 102 performance horses. AJTCVM 2014;9(2):33–41.
2. Lynn B. Cutaneous nociceptors. In: Winlow W, Holden AV, editors. The neurobiology of pain: symposium of the northern neurobiology group, held at leeds on 18 April 1983. Manchester (United Kingdom): Manchester University Press; 1984. p. 106.
3. Wiese AJ, Yaksh TL. Nociception and Pain Mechanisms. In: Handbook of Veterinary Pain Management. Third Edition. St Louis (IL): Elsevier; 2015. p. 10–41.
4. Vernon H, Aker P, Burns S, et al. Pressure pain threshold evaluation of the effect of spinal manipulation in the treatment of chronic neck pain: a pilot study. J Manipulative Physiol Ther 1990;13:13–6.
5. Kandel ER, Schwartz JH, Jessell TM, et al. McGraw-Hill Education/Medical; 5th edition (October 26, 2012), USA.
6. Xie H, Colahan P, Ott EA. Evaluation of electroacupuncture treatment of horses with signs of chronic thoracolumbar pain. J Am Vet Med Assoc 2005;227(2): 281–6.
7. Rungsri P, Trinarong C, Rojanasthien S, et al. Effectiveness of electro-acupuncture on pain threshold in sport horses with back pain. Am J Trad Chinese Vet Med 2009;4:22–6.
8. Song D, Xie H. Annotated Yuan Heng's classical collection on the treatment of equine diseases. Beijing: China Agriculture Press; 2012. p. 5–6.

9. Jaggar D, Robinson N. History of veterinary acupuncture. In: Schoen AM, editor. Veterinary acupuncture- ancient art to modern medicine. 2nd edition. St Louis (MO): Mosby; 2001. p. 7–9.
10. Memon MA, Sprunger LK. Survey of colleges and schools of veterinary medicine regarding education in complementary and alternative veterinary medicine. J Am Vet Med Assoc 2011;239:619–23.
11. Juan IJ, Wang Q, Liang H, et al. Biophysical characteristics of meridians and acupoints: a systematic review. Evid Based Complement Alternat Med 2012;2012: 793841.
12. Mense S, Simons DG. Muscle pain: understanding its nature, diagnosis and treatment. Philadelphia: Lippincott Williams & Wilkens; 2001.
13. Ma YT, Ma M, Cho ZH. Dynamic pathophysiology of acupoints. In: Biomedical acupuncture for pain management. St Louis (IL): Elsevier; 2005. p. 17–23.
14. Melzack R, Stillwell DM, Fox EJ. Trigger points and acupuncture points for pain: correlations and implications. Pain 1977;3:3–23.
15. Wang JW, Dong W, Wang C, et al. From meridians and acupoints to self-supervision and control system: a hypothesis of the 10th functional system based on anatomical studies of digitized virtual human. Nan Fang Yi Ke Da Xue Xue Bao 2007;27(5):573–9.
16. Langevin HM, Yandow JA. Relationship of acupuncture points and meridians to connective tissue planes. Anat Rec 2002;269(6):257–65.
17. Bai Y, Yuan L, Soh KS, et al. Possible applications for fascial anatomy and fasciaology in traditional chinese medicine. J Acupunct Meridian Stud 2010;3(2): 125–32.
18. Ma YT, Ma M, Cho ZH. From neurons to acupoints: basic neuroanatomy of acupoints. In: Biomedical acupuncture for pain management. St Louis (IL): Elsevier; 2005. p. 1–16.
19. Ma YT, Ma M, Cho ZH. Peripheral mechanisms of acupuncture. In: Biomedical acupuncture for pain management. St Louis (IL): Elsevier; 2005. p. 24–36.
20. Pomeranz B. Acupuncture analgesia - basic research. In: Stux G, Hammerschlag R, editors. Clinical acupuncture: scientific basis. Berlin: Springer; 2001. p. 1–28.
21. Julias M, Edgar LT, Buetttner HM, et al. An in vitro assay of collagen fiber alignment by acupuncture needle rotation. Biomed Eng Online 2008;7:19. Available at: http://biomedical-engineering-online.com/content/7/1/19.
22. Langevin HM, Konfagou EE, Badger GJ, et al. Tissue displacements during acupuncture using ultrasound elastography techniques. Ultrasound Med Biol 2004;30(9):1173–83.
23. Fox JR, Gray W, Koptiuch C, et al. Anisotropic tissue motion induced by acupuncture needling along intermuscular connective tissue planes. J Altern Complement Med 2014;20(4):290–4.
24. Schliep R, Jäger H, Klinger W. Fascia is alive: how cells modulate the tonicity and architecture of fascial tissues. In: Schliep R, Findlay TW, Chaitow L, et al, editors. Fascia: the tensional network of the human body. Edinburgh (Scotland): Churchill Livingstone Elsevier; 2012. p. 157–64.
25. Kumka M, Bonar J. Fascia: a morphological description and classification system based on a literature review. J Can Chiropr Assoc 2012;56(3):179–91.
26. Kwong EH, Findley TW. Fascia - current knowledge and future directions in physiatry: narrative review. J Rehabil Res Dev 2014;51(6):875–84.
27. Jiang XM, Zhang XQ, Yuan L. Advances in the study on the role of connective tissue in the mechanical signal transduction of acupuncture. Zhen Ci Yan Jiu 2009;34(2):136–9.

28. Wilke J, Krause F, Vogt L, et al. What is evidence-based about myofascial chains? a systemic review. Arch Phys Med Rehabil 2015. http://dx.doi.org/10.1016/j.apmr.2015.07.023.

29. Myers TW. Anatomy trains: myofascial meridians for manual and movement therapists. 3rd edition. Edinburgh (Scotland): Churchill Livingstone Elsevier; 2014.

30. Elbrønd VS, Schultz RM. Myofascial Kinetic Lines in Horses. Equine Veterinary Journal. 46:40. http://dx.doi.org/10.1111/evj.12267_121.

31. Goldman N, Chen M, Fujita T, et al. Adenosine A1 receptors mediate local antinociceptive effects of acupuncture. Nat Neurosci 2010;13(7):883088.

32. Langevin HM, Bouffard NA, Badger GJ, et al. Dynamic fibroblast cytoskeletal response to subcutaneous tissue stretch ex vivo and in vivo. Am J Physiol Cell Physiol 2005;288:C747–56.

33. Langevin HM, Bouffard NA, Churchill DL, et al. Connective tissue fibroblast response to acupuncture: dose-dependent effect of bidirectional needle rotation. J Altern Complement Med 2007;13(3):355–60.

34. Langevin HM, Fujita T, Bouffard NA, et al. Fibroblast cytoskeletal remodeling induced by tissue stretch involve ATP signaling. J Cell Physiol 2013;228(9):1922–6.

35. Takahashi M, Hoshino H, Kushida K, et al. Direct measurement of crosslinks, pyridinoline, deoxypyridinoline, and pentosidine, in the hydrolysate of tissues using high-performance liquid chromatography. Anal Biochem 1995;232:158–62.

36. Mays PK, McAnulty RJ, Campa RJ, et al. Age-related alerations in collagen and total protein metabolism determined in cultured rat dermal fibroblasts: age-related trends parallel those observed in rat skin in vivo. Int J Biochem Cell Biol 1995;27(9):937–45.

37. Geng X, Sun T, Li JH, et al. Electroacupuncture in the repair of spinal cord injury: inhibiting the notch signaling pathway and promoting neural stem cell proliferation. Neural Regen Res 2015;10(3):394–403.

38. Xiao Y, Wu X, Deng X, et al. Optimal electroacupuncture frequency for maintaining astrocyte structural integrity in cerebral ischemia. Neural Regen Res 2013;8(12):1122–31.

39. He GH, Ruan JW, Zeng YS, et al. Improvement in acupoint selection for acupuncture of nerves surrounding the injury site: electro-acupuncture with governor vessel with local meridian acupoints. Neural Regen Res 2015;10(1):128–35.

40. May K. Equine Acupuncture – Acupuncture Points and Meridians (Channels). In: Certification Course in Basic Veterinary Acupuncture Course Notes – Portland (OR). 24th edition. Fort Collins (CO): The International Veterinary Acupuncture Society (IVAS); 2014. p. 131–68.

41. Hwang Y-C, Yu C. Traditional equine acupuncture atlas. In: Schoen AM, editor. Veterinary acupuncture – ancient art to modern medicine. 2nd edition. St Louis (MO): Mosby; 2001. p. 363–91.

42. Fleming P. Traditional equine acupuncture atlas. In: Schoen AM, editor. Veterinary acupuncture – ancient art to modern medicine. 2nd edition. St Louis (MO): Mosby; 2001. p. 393–431.

43. May K. Use of Acupuncture in the treatment of equine neurological problems. The 10th Annual Canadian Oriental Medical Symposium. Vancouver, BC, March 14, 2013.

44. May K. Use of acupuncture for diagnosis and treatment of sore backs in equine – even in the most reluctant cases. In: Knueven D, editor. Proceedings for Annual Conference of the American Holistic Veterinary Medical Association. Abingdon

(MD): American Holistic Veterinary Medical Association. San Diego; 2011. p. 231–4.

45. May K. Equine neck pain using both traditional and transpositional meridian and non-meridian acupuncture points. In: Knueven D, editor. Proceedings for Annual Conference of the American Holistic Veterinary Medical Association. Abingdon (MD): American Holistic Veterinary Medical Association. San Diego; 2011. p. 235–8.

46. May K. Equine traditional, transpositional and non-meridian points – a comparison of location and use and palpation tips. In: Knueven D, editor. Proceedings for Annual Conference of the American Holistic Veterinary Medical Association. Abingdon (MD): American Holistic Veterinary Medical Association. San Diego; 2011. p. 239–68.

Joint Mobilization and Manipulation for the Equine Athlete

Kevin K. Haussler, DVM, DC, PhD

KEYWORDS

- Equine • Joint mobilization • Manipulation • Rehabilitation • Back pain
- Manual therapy

KEY POINTS

- Joint mobilization and manipulation provide important diagnostic and therapeutic approaches for addressing musculoskeletal issues in equine sports medicine and rehabilitation.
- Soft tissue mobilization focuses on restoring movement to the skin, connective tissue, ligaments, tendons, and muscles with the goal of modulating pain, reducing inflammation, improving tissue repair, increasing extensibility, and improving function.
- Joint mobilization is characterized as nonimpulsive, repetitive joint movements induced within the passive range of joint motion with the purpose of restoring normal and symmetric joint range of motion, to stretch connective tissues, and to restore normal joint end-feel.
- Manipulation is a manual procedure that involves a directed impulse that moves a joint or vertebral segment beyond its physiologic range of motion.
- A thorough knowledge of equine anatomy, soft tissue and joint biomechanics, musculoskeletal pathology, and tissue-healing processes is required to apply joint mobilization and manipulation techniques.

INTRODUCTION

Joint mobilization and manipulation are considered forms of manual therapy, which involves the application of the hands to the body with a therapeutic intent.[1] Soft tissue mobilization focuses on restoring movement to the skin, connective tissue, ligaments, tendons, and muscles with the goal of modulating pain, reducing inflammation, improving tissue repair, increasing extensibility, and improving function.[2] Joint mobilization is characterized as nonimpulsive, repetitive joint movements induced within the passive range of joint motion with the purpose of restoring normal and symmetric joint range of motion, to stretch connective tissues, and to restore normal joint end-feel.[3] Manipulation is a manual procedure that involves a directed impulse that moves

Department of Clinical Sciences, Gail Holmes Equine Orthopaedic Research Center, College of Veterinary Medicine and Biomedical Sciences, Colorado State University, 300 West Drake Road, Fort Collins, CO 80523, USA

E-mail address: Kevin.Haussler@ColoState.edu

Vet Clin Equine 32 (2016) 87–101
http://dx.doi.org/10.1016/j.cveq.2015.12.003
0749-0739/16/$ – see front matter © 2016 Published by Elsevier Inc.

a joint or vertebral segment beyond its physiologic range of motion, but does not exceed the anatomic limit of the articulation.[4] The primary biomechanical difference between joint mobilization and manipulation is the presence of a high-speed thrust or impulse. Spinal manipulation involves the application of controlled impulses to articular structures within the axial skeleton with the intent of reducing pain and muscle hypertonicity and increasing joint range of motion.[5]

OBJECTIVES OF TREATMENT

All rehabilitation programs should be established based on individual patient needs and disabilities. General categories of rehabilitation issues that need to be assessed in every patient include pain, proprioception, flexibility, endurance, and strength. Each of these rehabilitation issues then need to have specific, detailed treatment plans developed with objective endpoints and outcome measures to identify accomplishment of each treatment goal. Soft tissue and joint mobilization are used to assess the quality and quantity of joint range of motion and as a primary means of treating musculoskeletal disorders. Subjective assessment of the ease of joint motion, joint stability, and joint end-feel provide insights into the biomechanical and neurologic features of an articulation. Goniometry is often used to objectively quantify and document the amount of flexion or extension present at an articulation.[6] The objectives of soft tissue and joint mobilization are typically to reduce pain, restore tissue compliance, and to improve overall tissue mobility and joint range of motion.[2] Manipulation is more often used to address localized pain and joint stiffness, with less focus on the surrounding soft tissues.[5] Manual therapy techniques can also provide an adjunct to therapeutic exercises and rehabilitation of neuromotor control, where applied forces are used to induce passive stretching, weight-shifting and activation of spinal reflexes, which help to increase flexibility, stimulate proprioception, and strengthen core musculature.[7] Peripheral nerve and nerve root mobilization techniques and exercises are also used for postoperative rehabilitation of low back pain.[8] Few formal studies exist to support the use of active joint or spinal mobilization techniques in horses.[9] Most mobilization studies in horses involve a period of induced joint immobilization by a fixture or cast followed by allowing the horse to spontaneously weight bear and locomote on the affected limb, without evaluation of specific soft tissue or joint-mobilization techniques.[10]

JOINT MECHANICS

The use of palpation techniques to qualitatively and quantitatively assess joint motion requires an understanding of joint mechanics.[11] Joint motion can be categorized into 3 zones of movement: physiologic, paraphysiologic, and pathologic (**Fig. 1**). The

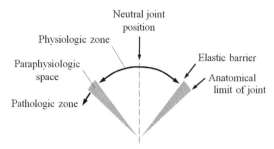

Fig. 1. Graphic representation of joint mechanics as they relate to the zones of joint motion.

physiologic zone of movement consists of both active and passive joint motion within all possible directions of movement (eg, flexion, extension, lateral bending, and axial rotation). Passive movement of an articulation from a neutral joint position first involves evaluating the range of joint motion that has minimal, uniform resistance. Then, as the articulation is moved toward the end range of passive joint motion, there is a gradual increase in the resistance to movement, which terminates at an elastic barrier (ie, joint end-feel). The end range of motion begins with any palpable change in resistance to passive joint mobilization. Joint end-feel is often evaluated by bringing an individual articulation to tension and applying rhythmic oscillations to qualify the resistance to movement.[12] Normal joint end-feel is initially soft and resilient and gradually becomes more restrictive as the limits of joint range of motion are reached. A pathologic or restrictive end range of motion is palpable earlier in passive joint movement and has an abrupt, hard end-feel when compared with normal joint end-feel. Each articulation within the body has unique palpatory end-feels for each of the directions of joint motion (eg, flexion, extension, lateral bending). The goal of palpating passive joint movement is to evaluate each articulation of interest for quality of joint motion, the initiation of resistance to motion and type of end-feel, and the amount of motion within each of the principal directions of movement. The paraphysiologic space is bordered by the elastic and anatomic limits of an individual joint. Joint motion into the paraphysiologic space occurs only with the application of high-velocity forces associated with joint manipulation. The anatomic barrier of the joint marks the junction between the paraphysiologic and pathologic zones of movement. The pathologic zone is characterized by the application of excessive forces or joint motion that causes an articulation to move beyond its anatomic limits and results in mechanical disruption of intra-articular and periarticular structures and subsequent joint instability or luxation.

Active range of motion is characterized by the amplitude of voluntary joint movements (eg, flexion and extension) produced by active muscle contractions (**Fig. 2**). Vertebral range of motion in left and right lateral bending or axial rotation is typically distributed symmetrically about a neutral joint position; however, joint ranges of motion in flexion versus extension at certain vertebral levels or limb articulations may be quite asymmetrical.[13,14] Passive joint range of motion can be assessed only with the application of external articular forces. The limit of passive joint motion occurs beyond the range of voluntary joint movements and is the site where joint mobilization and stretching exercises are applied (**Fig. 3**). Joint mobilization and manipulation are 2 types of induced articular movements used in musculoskeletal rehabilitation to restore joint mobility and reduce pain. Mobilization is characterized as repetitive joint movements induced within the normal physiologic range of joint motion. Joint manipulation involves the application of force to bring an articulation to end range of motion

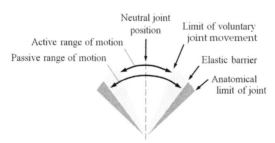

Fig. 2. Graphic representation of joint mechanics as they relate to the active and passive joint ranges of motion.

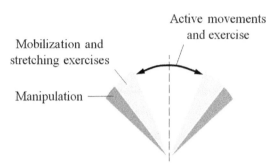

Fig. 3. Graphic representation of joint mechanics as they relate to sites of active joint movement, joint mobilization, and manipulation.

(ie, pretension) and then applying a thrust or impulse to move the joint of interest beyond the elastic barrier and into the paraphysiologic zone with the intent of stimulating both mechanical and neurophysiologic mechanisms.

MECHANISMS OF ACTION

Joint mobilization and manipulation produce physiologic effects within local tissues, on sensory and motor components of the nervous system, and at a psychological or behavioral level.[1] It is likely that specific manual therapy techniques are inherently more effective than others in addressing each of these local, regional, or systemic components.[15] The challenge is in choosing the most appropriate form of joint mobilization or manipulation or combination of techniques that will be efficacious for an individual patient with specific musculoskeletal disabilities. If soft tissue restriction and pain are identified as the primary components of a musculoskeletal injury, then massage, stretching, and soft tissue mobilization techniques are indicated for increasing tissue extensibility.[16] However, if the musculoskeletal dysfunction is localized to articular structures, then stretching, joint mobilization, and manipulation are the most indicated manual therapy techniques for restoring joint range of motion and reducing pain.[17]

Local tissue effects produced by joint mobilization and manipulation techniques relate to direct mechanical stimulation of skin, fascia, muscles, tendons, ligaments, and joint capsules.[18] Mechanical effects also can influence the vasculature, lymphatics, and synovial fluid.[19] Direct mechanical loading of tissues can alter tissue healing, the physical properties of tissues (eg, elongation), and local tissue fluid dynamics associated with extracellular or intravascular fluids. Normal tissue repair and remodeling rely on mechanical stimulation of cells and tissues to restore optimal structural and functional properties, such as tensile strength and flexibility. Nonspecific back pain is most likely related to a functional impairment and not a structural disorder; therefore, many back problems may be related to muscle or joint dysfunction with secondary soft tissue irritation and pain generation.[11] Soft tissue contractures and adhesions are unwanted effects associated with musculoskeletal injuries and postsurgical immobilization.[10] Stretching exercises or direct mechanical mobilization of the affected tissue can be used to elongate contracted or fibrotic connective tissues to improve soft tissue extensibility and increase joint range of motion.[16] Tissue viability is highly dependent on its vascular and lymphatic supply, which is often compromised due to mechanical disruption or ischemia. Soft tissue or joint mobilization may facilitate flow to and from the affected tissues, help to reduce pain and edema, and decrease joint effusion.[19] Joint manipulation can improve restricted joint mobility and may reduce the harmful effects associated with joint immobilization and joint capsule contractures. Limb and joint mobilization also can have direct mechanical effects on nerve roots and the dura mater, which may have clinical application in the treatment of perineural adhesions and edema.[20]

Soft tissue manipulation has the additional effect of stimulating regional or systemic changes in neurologic signaling related to pain processing and motor control. Joint mobilization and manipulation can provide effective management of pain and neuromuscular deficits associated with musculoskeletal injuries, alterations in postural control, and locomotory issues related to antalgic or compensatory gait.[1] In response to chronic pain or stiffness, new movement patterns are developed by the nervous system and adopted in an attempt to reduce pain or discomfort. Long after the initial injury has healed, adaptive or secondary movement patterns may continue to persist, which predispose adjacent articulations or muscles to injury.[11] Activation of proprioceptors, nociceptors, and components of the muscle spindles provide afferent stimuli that have direct and widespread influences on components of the peripheral and central nervous systems that directly regulate muscle tone and movement patterns.[11] The various forms of manual therapy are thought to affect different aspects of joint function via diverse mechanical and neurologic mechanisms.[21] Alterations in articular neurophysiology from mechanical or chemical injuries can affect both mechanoreceptor and nociceptor function via increased joint capsule tension and nerve-ending hypersensitivity.[22] Mechanoreceptor stimulation induces reflex paraspinal musculature hypertonicity and altered local and systemic neurologic reflexes. Nociceptor stimulation results in a lowered pain threshold, sustained afferent stimulation (ie, facilitation), reflex paraspinal musculature hypertonicity, and abnormal neurologic reflexes. Touch and light massage preferentially stimulate superficial proprioceptors, whereas any technique that involves deep tissue massage, stretching, muscle contraction, or joint movement has the potential to stimulate deep proprioceptors.[1] Massage, stretching, and joint mobilization are also considered to affect more superficial epaxial muscles, such as the longissimus muscle, and to have a multisegmental effect. In contrast, manipulation preferentially stimulates mechanoreceptors within deep multifidi muscles and has a more segmental focus.[23] Joint manipulation can affect mechanoreceptors (ie, Golgi tendon organ and muscle spindles) to induce reflex inhibition of pain and muscle relaxation and to correct abnormal movement patterns.[24] Due to somatovisceral innervation, mobilization and manipulation within the trunk have possible influences on the autonomic system and visceral functions; however, the clinical significance and repeatability of these effects are largely unknown.[25]

CLINICAL INDICATIONS

Joint mobilization and manipulation provide important diagnostic and therapeutic approaches for addressing equine axial skeleton problems that are not otherwise available in veterinary medicine. Most of the current knowledge about equine manual therapies has been borrowed from human techniques, theories, and research and applied to horses. Therapeutic trials of joint mobilization or manipulation are often used because of limited knowledge about the effects of manual therapy in horses. The indications for joint mobilization and manipulation are similar and include restricted joint range of motion, muscle spasms, pain, fibrosis, or contracted soft tissues.[3] The principal indications for spinal manipulation are neck or back pain, localized or regional joint stiffness, poor performance, and altered gait that is not associated with overt lameness. A thorough diagnostic workup is required to identify soft tissue and osseous pathology, neurologic disorders, or other lameness conditions that may not be responsive to manual therapy. Clinical signs indicative of a primary spinal disorder include localized musculoskeletal pain, muscle hypertonicity, and restricted joint motion. This triad of clinical signs also can be found in a variety of lower limb disorders; however, they are most evident in horses with neck or back problems. Clinical signs indicative of chronic or secondary spinal disorders include regional or diffuse pain, generalized stiffness, and widespread muscle hypertonicity. In these cases, further diagnostic evaluation or imaging should be done to identify the primary cause of lameness or poor performance.

Joint mobilization and manipulation are critical components in the management of muscular, articular, and neurologic components of select musculoskeletal injuries in performance horses. Musculoskeletal conditions that are chronic or recurring, not readily diagnosed, or are not responding to conventional veterinary care may be indicators that manual therapy evaluation and treatment are needed. Joint mobilization and manipulation are typically more effective in the early clinical stages of disease processes versus end-stage disease, where reparative processes have been exhausted. Joint manipulation is usually contraindicated in the acute stages of soft tissue injury; however, mobilization is safer than manipulation and has been shown to have short-term benefits for acute neck or back pain in humans.[26] Manipulation is probably more effective than mobilization for chronic neck or back pain and has the potential to help restore normal joint motion, thus limiting the risk of reinjury.[11] It has been theorized that spinal manipulation preferentially influences a sensory bed, which, in terms of anatomic location and function, is different from the sensory bed influenced by spinal mobilization techniques.[23] Manipulation may preferentially stimulate receptors within deep intervertebral muscles, whereas mobilization techniques most likely affect more superficial axial muscles. Only one study has compared mobilization with manipulation in horses, and spinal manipulation induced a 15% increase in displacement and a 20% increase in applied force, compared with mobilization.[9] At most vertebral sites studied, manipulation increased the amplitudes of dorsoventral displacement and applied force, indicative of increased spinal flexibility and increased tolerance to pressure in the thoracolumbar region of the equine vertebral column.

ACTIVE AND PASSIVE STRETCHING EXERCISES

Stretching exercises vary according to the direction, velocity, amplitude, and duration of the applied force or induced movement. However, it is difficult to identify which combination of positions, techniques, and durations of stretching are the most effective to induce increased joint range of motion.[27] Active stretching involves using the patient's own movements to induce a stretch, whereas passive stretches are applied to relaxed muscles or connective tissues during passive soft tissue or joint mobilization. In horses, active stretches of the neck and trunk are often induced with baited (ie, carrot) stretches with the goal in increasing flexion, extension, or lateral bending of the axial skeleton. Asking horses to produce active stretching of the limbs is often difficult; therefore, passive stretches are most commonly prescribed in horses.[28] Stretching should be performed slowly to maximize tissue elongation due to creep and stress relaxation within fibrotic or shortened periarticular soft tissues.[16] Sustained, low-load stretching is more effective than rapid, high-load stretching for altering viscoelastic properties within soft tissues.[29] Rapid stretching may exceed the tissue's mechanical properties and produce additional trauma within injured tissues.[30] The force applied during stretching exercises should be tailored to specific phases of tissue repair.[16] During the acute inflammatory phase, stretching should be mostly avoided because of the increased risk of tissue injury. During the regenerative and remodeling phases of healing, tissues progressively regain tensile strength, and applied manual forces can be gradually increased. The amount of force applied during passive stretching is largely based on the patient's response and signs of pain. Musculoskeletal injuries are characterized by multiple tissue involvement, each of which has a different healing rate and unique mechanical response to stretching. Therefore, effective stretching programs are best tailored to address specific soft tissue injuries and not only focused on restoring joint motion.

Passive stretching consists of applying forces to a limb or body segment so as to lengthen muscles or connective tissues beyond their normal resting lengths, with the intent of increasing joint range of motion and flexibility.[31] The amplitude of motion and length of time that an individual stretch is held is gradually increased over time according to patient tolerance and ability. In horses, passive stretching exercises of the limbs and axial skeleton have anecdotal effects of increasing stride length and joint range of motion and improving overall comfort.[28] In a noncontrolled study, passive thoracic limb stretching lowered wither height due to possible relaxation of the fibromuscular thoracic girdle.[32] However, a randomized controlled trial in riding school horses evaluating the effect of 2 different 8-week passive stretching programs reported no significant changes in stride length at the trot but actual decreases in joint range of motion within the shoulder, stifle, and hock articulations.[33] The investigators concluded that daily stretching may be too intensive in normal horses and may actually cause negative biomechanical effects. Additional studies on the effects of different stretching techniques and frequency for specific disease processes using objective outcome measures need to be completed before any further claims of performance enhancement in horses can be made.

The duration of the applied stretch is dependent on the force applied, affected tissue shape and size, the amount of damage or fibrosis present, and the stage of tissue healing.[16] In humans, the recommended duration for stretching the musculotendinous unit varies from 6 to 60 seconds.[30] Stretching for 30 seconds has been shown to be significantly more effective than 15-second stretches; however, structural and functional differences within each affected tissue make general recommendations for stretching a particular articulation or limb difficult to establish.[34] The mode of loading during an applied stretch varies from continuous to cyclic. Continuous or static loading during stretching exercises can be uncomfortable for some patients and is not recommended.[16] Cyclic or rhythmic stretching is more comfortable and physiologic, as it provides periods of tissue loading and unloading, which has biomechanical and neurologic benefits. Cyclic loading also has cumulative effects on soft tissues due to incremental elongation and stress relaxation within each stretch cycle; however, these effects are maximized approximately within the first 4 cycles of loading.[30] Therefore, recommendations for optimal passive stretching include applying 4 to 5 repetitions of slow, low-load forces held at the end range of motion of the affected tissues, with each stretch applied and released in 30-second cycles, without inducing pain. If performed inappropriately, stretches may cause or aggravate injuries.[35] Therefore, thorough patient evaluation and proper stretching program design are required before implementing stretches. With minimal training, horses and their owners can be taught how to do simple but effective passive joint mobilization and active stretching exercises (ie, carrot stretches) to improve both limb and axial skeleton flexibility.

JOINT MOBILIZATION AND MANIPULATION TECHNIQUES

Selection factors for considering mobilization versus manipulation include the technical training and skill of the practitioner, perceived risks versus benefits, the presence of acute pain and inflammation, and pathoanatomic considerations.[23] Joint mobilization is easier to apply, requires fewer psychomotor skills, has minimal risks, and can be used in the presence of acute pain and inflammation, compared with manipulation. Manual therapy procedures are also dependent on the ability of the patient to relax and the patent response to the applied force. Characteristics of joint mobilization and manipulation include factors related to specificity, leverage, velocity, amplitude, direction, and prestress of the applied force.[21] Additional factors are related to joint position and frequency or oscillation of the applied forces.[3] Levers are used to increase mechanical advantage and assist in applying force to an articulation or body segment to induce joint motion. Long levers include using the limbs or head and neck as levers to induce spinal motion, instead of the inducing motion at 1 or 2 individual vertebrae by using transverse or spinous processes as short lever contacts. Velocity relates to the speed of the impulse applied to move a vertebra or body segment and displacement is the distance over which the applied thrust is applied. Amplitude refers to the amount of force applied. With long-lever techniques, lower amplitudes of force are required to induce similar joint motion as short-lever contacts. However, the rationale for using short-lever techniques is to increase the specificity of the applied thrust, as a single vertebral process is contacted on the vertebra of interest with short-lever techniques. With long levers, it is likely that multiple articulations are included between the doctor's contact and the body segment of interest, which produces a more generalized treatment effect. Using a specific contact is theorized to address a single articulation; however, studies on treatment effects indicate that specific contact techniques produce local, as well as regional and systemic effects.[36] The therapeutic dosage of joint mobilization or manipulation is also determined by the number of vertebrae or body segments treated and the frequency of the applied treatments.

Biomechanical characteristics of joint mobilization include low peak forces, slow application, low-velocity movements, and large displacements. Mobilization of the thoracic spine produces 2-cm to 3-cm displacements, whereas manipulation induces 6-mm to 12-mm displacements.[23] Mobilization is typically applied with long-lever arm, low-velocity, oscillatory forces within or at the limits of physiologic joint range of motion without imparting a thrust or impulse. Mobilization also is performed within the patient's ability to resist the applied motion and therefore requires cooperation and relaxation of the patient. Mobilization is usually applied in a graded manner, with each grade increasing the range of joint movement. Grades 1 and 2 mobilizations are characterized by slow oscillations within the first 25% to 50% of the available joint motion, with the goal of reducing pain. Grades 3 and 4 mobilizations involve slow oscillations at or near the end of available joint motion, which are used to increase joint range of motion. Some mobilization techniques may include a hold and stretch at the end range of motion. Distraction or traction refers to applying manual or mechanical forces to induce separation of adjacent joint surfaces, which causes stretching of the joint capsule, reduced intra-articular pressure, and is often used to reduce joint luxations.

Manipulation is characterized by short-lever arm, high-velocity, low-amplitude forces applied outside of the physiologic zone of joint motion. Therefore, it is often difficult for patients to resist or guard against the applied impulse. Chiropractic techniques are often characterized as high-velocity, low-amplitude thrusts delivered to a specified vertebral process (short-lever arm) in a specific direction.[21] Osteopathic techniques also include similar high-velocity, low-amplitude thrusts applied to single or multiple articulations with the goal of increasing joint range of motion and reducing pain.[37] Mobilization and manipulation forces can both be focused on a specific joint or anatomic region in a specific direction; however, mobilization is often considered a general technique and manipulation is theoretically considered more specific. The therapeutic dosage of applied mobilizations or manipulations is modified by the number of vertebrae or articulations treated, the amount of force applied, and the frequency and duration of treatment. Unfortunately, there is not good scientific evidence on which to base optimal dosage recommendations for continued care; therefore, therapeutic trials are often used on an individual basis.[38] The goal of manual therapy is to restore normal joint motion, stimulate neurologic reflexes, and reduce pain and muscle hypertonicity. Comparisons of sensitivity to palpation, muscle tone, and joint motion are made before and after treatment to evaluate the response to and effectiveness of manual therapy.

Anecdotal evidence and clinical experience suggest that manipulation is an effective adjunctive modality for the conservative treatment of select musculoskeletal-related disorders in horses.[39] Therapeutic trials of spinal manipulation are often used, because there is currently limited formal research available about the effectiveness of osteopathic or chiropractic techniques in equine practice. Equine osteopathic evaluation and treatment procedures have been described in textbooks and case reports, but no formal hypothesis-driven research exists.[37,40,41] The focus of recent equine chiropractic research has been on assessing the clinical effects of spinal manipulation on pain relief, improving flexibility, reducing muscle hypertonicity, and restoring spinal motion symmetry. Obvious criticism has been directed at the physical ability to even induce movement in the horse's back. Pilot work has demonstrated that manually applied forces associated with chiropractic techniques are able to produce substantial segmental spinal motion.[42] Two randomized, controlled clinical trials using pressure algometry to assess mechanical nociceptive thresholds (MNTs) in the thoracolumbar region of horses have demonstrated that both manual and instrument-assisted spinal manipulation can reduce back pain (or increase MNTs).[43,44] Additional studies have assessed the effects of equine chiropractic techniques on increasing passive spinal mobility (ie, flexibility) and reducing longissimus muscle tone.[9,45] The effect of manipulation on asymmetrical spinal movement patterns in horses with documented back pain suggest that chiropractic treatment elicits slight but significant changes in thoracolumbar and pelvic kinematics and that some of these changes are likely to be beneficial.[46,47]

MUSCULOSKELETAL EXAMINATION

A complete musculoskeletal examination includes assessment of active and passive joint ranges of motion for all axial and appendicular articulations of interest. Active joint range of motion of the axial skeleton is evaluated during normal daily activities (eg, lying to standing movements or locomotion) or during induced vertebral movements while using a carrot or other treat to produce active movements of the head, neck, or trunk. Similar procedures can be used therapeutically as active stretching exercises to increase neck or trunk range of motion or for developing coordination and strength of the muscles responsible for trunk stabilization.[7] Normal vertebral movements consist of varying amounts and combinations of flexion, extension, left and right lateral bending, and left and right axial rotation. Active joint motion within most equine limb articulations consists almost exclusively of flexion-extension, with occasional joints capable of undergoing small amounts of internal or external rotation. Abnormal active joint motion is characterized by weakness, incoordination, asymmetry, or restricted or excessive joint movements. The willingness, coordination, and amount of vertebral or limb segment motion is compared bilaterally and left-to-right range of motion asymmetries are documented. Local or regional causes of active vertebral movement restrictions or altered movement may include peripheral or central neuropathies, myopathies, intra-articular pathology (ie, osteoarthritis), periarticular soft tissue adhesions, musculotendinous contractures, or protective muscle spasms. Joint hypermobility is usually indicative of articular instability, which often requires immediate medical or surgical evaluation and stabilization and is generally a contraindication for most forms of manual therapy.

Passive joint range of motion is evaluated by measuring the amount and characteristics of joint motion beyond the active range of joint motion (see **Fig. 2**). Assessing passive range of motion requires patient cooperation and muscular relaxation, as each articulation is moved passively throughout its unique ranges and directions of motion. The goal of palpating joint movement is to evaluate the quality of joint motion, the initiation of resistance to motion and joint end-feel, and the amplitude of joint motion present. Similar palpatory findings can be identified in soft tissues, such as skin, connective tissue, muscles, or ligaments.[48] Passive joint range of motion is evaluated to detect whether a particular movement is normal, restricted, or hypermobile. Passive joint mobility can be assessed either segmentally via palpation of individual vertebral motion segments or limb articulations, or evaluated regionally via passive mobilization of vertebral regions or entire limbs. Causes of restricted articular movement include soft tissue (eg, capsular fibrosis, muscle spasms, or contractures) and osseous pathologies (eg, malformations, osteoarthritis, or ankylosis). Restricted vertebral segment motion can occur with or without localized muscle hypertonicity or pain. Diagnostic interpretations of joint function can be implied by combining evaluation of joint range of motion and pain at the extremes of joint motion.[49] Normal joint motion is painless, suggesting that articular structures are intact and functional. Normal joint mobility that has a painful end range of movement suggests a minor sprain of periarticular tissues or muscle. Painless joint hypomobility suggests a soft tissue contracture or adhesion. Painful joint hypomobility suggests an acute strain or intra-articular injury with secondary muscle guarding. Painless hypermobility of an articulation may indicate a complete rupture, whereas painful hypermobility suggests a partial tear of an intra-articular or periarticular structure.

Evaluation of passive joint range of motion within the axial skeleton begins at the head and continues to the tip of the tail. In a relaxed horse, left-right lateral excursion of the mandible is assessed for amplitude, quality, and symmetry.[50] Palpation of mandibular range of motion and audible contact of the incisors and cheek teeth are compared bilaterally. The dorsal and lateral excursion of the lingual process and basihyoid bone of the hyoid apparatus is assessed for restricted motion and pain, indicative of possible temporohyoid osteoarthropathy. The occipitoatlantal (Occ–C1) articulation is evaluated in full ranges of flexion, extension, and lateral bending for signs of pain or resisted motion. The atlantoaxial (C1–C2) articulation is evaluated for altered or asymmetrical ranges of axial rotation. The intervertebral articulations of the second to seventh cervical vertebrae (C2–C7) are assessed individually for altered joint range of motion and joint end-feel during combined lateral bending and rotation.[50] Articulations of the mid-cervical region (C4–C6) are commonly restricted and painful in performance horses, presumably because of locally altered biomechanical influences. The individual spinous processes of the third to twelfth thoracic vertebrae (T3–T12) are manually deviated from midline, while monitoring for signs of reduced vertebral motion, localized or generalized pain response, and induced muscle hypertonicity.[51] Horses with poorly fitting saddles (ie, tree is too narrow) resent palpation and passive motion of the affected cranial thoracic vertebrae. The remaining thoracolumbar region (T13–L6) is evaluated in lateral bending and flexion and extension for similar signs of spinal dysfunction. Normal lateral bending range of motion is maximal at the mid-thoracic region and gradually diminishes toward the lumbosacral junction.[14] Conversely, flexion and extension are minimal within the thoracic region and gradually increase toward the lumbosacral junction, which is the site of maximal flexion and extension range of motion. Evaluation of segmental vertebral motion in flexion and extension requires the clinician to be on an elevated surface to induce ventrally directed rhythmic oscillations over the individual thoracolumbar intervertebral articulations. Horses with impinged dorsal spinous processes strongly resent any induced extension of the affected vertebral segments. The pelvis and sacroiliac joints are evaluated for motion restrictions and pain during induced joint motion with directed ventrally forces applied over the tuber coxae or during abaxial compression of the tubera sacrale.[50] The caudal vertebrae are assessed by passive range of motion of each intervertebral articulation and by applying axial traction to the tail. The passive range of motion of all thoracic and pelvic limb articulations are also evaluated in flexion and extension, internal and external rotation, abduction and adduction, and circumduction for signs of restricted joint motion, pain, inflammation, and muscle hypertonicity. Comparisons of the quality and quantity of passive range of motion are evaluated before and after stretching exercises or joint manipulation to assess potential therapeutic responses within limb articulations or vertebral motion segments.[52]

CONTRAINDICATIONS

Contraindications for joint mobilization and manipulation are often based on clinical judgment and are related to the technique applied and skill or experience of the practitioner.[3] Few absolute contraindications exist for joint mobilization if techniques are applied appropriately. Manual therapy is not a "cure-all" for all joint or back problems and is generally contraindicated in the presence of fractures, acute inflammatory or infectious joint disease, osteomyelitis, joint ankylosis, bleeding disorders, progressive neurologic signs, and primary or metastatic tumors.[3] Joint mobilization and manipulation cannot reverse severe degenerative processes or overt pathology. Acute episodes of osteoarthritis, impinged dorsal spinous processes, and severe articular instability, such as joint subluxation or luxation, are often contraindications for manipulation. Inadequate physical or spinal examination and poorly developed manipulative skills are also contraindications for applying manual therapy.[53] All horses with neurologic diseases should be evaluated fully to assess the potential risks or benefits of joint mobilization or manipulation. Cervical vertebral myelopathy occurs because of both structural and functional disorders.[54] Static compression caused by vertebral malformation and dynamic lesions caused by vertebral segment hypermobility are contraindications for cervical manipulation; however, adjacent regions of hypomobile vertebrae may benefit from mobilization or manipulation to help restore joint motion and reduce biomechanical stresses in the affected vertebral segments. Serious diseases requiring immediate medical or surgical care need to be ruled out and treated by conventional veterinary medicine before any routine manual therapy is initiated, although manual techniques provide important tools in the rehabilitation of most postsurgical cases or severe musculoskeletal injuries by helping to restore normal joint motion and function. Horses that have concurrent hock pain (eg, osteoarthritis) and a stiff, painful thoracolumbar or lumbosacral vertebral region are best managed by addressing all areas of musculoskeletal dysfunction. A multidisciplinary approach entails combined medical treatment of the hock osteoarthritis and manual therapy evaluation and treatment of the back problem.

ADVERSE EFFECTS

In humans, adverse effects or risks of complications associated with joint mobilization are minimal. Mobilization is considered safer than manipulation.[26] In humans, most adverse events associated with spinal manipulation are benign and self-limiting.[55] Potential mild adverse effects from properly applied manipulations include transient stiffness or worsening of the condition after treatment. Data from prospective studies suggest that minor, transient adverse events occur in approximately half of all patients during a course of spinal manipulative therapy; however, these mild adverse effects do not cause patients to stop seeking manipulative care.[56,57] Mild adverse effects usually last fewer than 1 to 2 days and resolve without concurrent medical intervention. Even though the complication rate of spinal manipulation is small, the potential for adverse outcomes must be considered because of the possibility of permanent impairment or death.[26] The benefits of chiropractic care in humans seem to outweigh the potential risks.[58]

The risk of adverse effects associated with joint mobilization or spinal manipulation is unknown in horses. The apparent safety of spinal manipulation, especially when compared with other medically accepted treatments for neck or low back pain in humans, should stimulate its use in the conservative treatment of spinal-related problems.[59,60] If an exacerbation of musculoskeletal dysfunction or lameness is noted after spinal manipulation, then a thorough reexamination and appropriate medical treatment should be pursued. If the condition does not improve with conservative care, referral for more extensive diagnostic evaluation or more aggressive medical treatment is recommended.

REFERENCES

1. Lederman E. Fundamentals of manual therapy: physiology, neurology and psychology. St Louis (MO): Churchill Livingstone; 1997.
2. Bromiley MW. Massage techniques for horse and rider. Wiltshire (England): The Crowood Press Ltd; 2002.
3. Scaringe J, Kawaoka C. Mobilization techniques. In: Haldeman S, editor. Principles and practice of chiropractic. 3rd edition. New York: McGraw-Hill; 2005. p. 767–85.
4. Gatterman MI. What's in a word. In: Gatterman MI, editor. Foundations of chiropractic. St Louis (MO): Mosby-Year Book, Inc; 1995. p. 5–17.
5. Haussler KK. Chiropractic evaluation and management. Vet Clin North Am Equine Pract 1999;15:195–209.
6. Liljebrink Y, Bergh A. Goniometry: is it a reliable tool to monitor passive joint range of motion in horses? Equine Vet J 2010;42(Suppl 38):676–82.
7. Stubbs NC, Clayton HM. Activate your horse's core: unmounted exercises for dynamic mobility, strength and balance. Mason (MI): Sport Horse Publications; 2008.
8. Ellis RF, Hing WA. Neural mobilization: a systematic review of randomized controlled trials with an analysis of therapeutic efficacy. J Man Manip Ther 2008;16:8–22.
9. Haussler KK, Hill AE, Puttlitz CM, et al. Effects of vertebral mobilization and manipulation on kinematics of the thoracolumbar region. Am J Vet Res 2007; 68:508–16.

10. van Harreveld PD, Lillich JD, Kawcak CE, et al. Clinical evaluation of the effects of immobilization followed by remobilization and exercise on the metacarpophalangeal joint in horses. Am J Vet Res 2002;63:282–8.

11. Liebenson C. Rehabilitation of the spine. 1st edition. Baltimore (MD): Williams & Wilkins; 1996.

12. Haneline MT, Cooperstein R, Young M, et al. Spinal motion palpation: a comparison of studies that assessed intersegmental end feel vs excursion. J Manipulative Physiol Ther 2008;31:616–26.

13. Clayton HM, Townsend HG. Kinematics of the cervical spine of the adult horse. Equine Vet J 1989;21:189–92.

14. Townsend HG, Leach DH, Fretz PB. Kinematics of the equine thoracolumbar spine. Equine Vet J 1983;15:117–22.

15. Triano J. The theoretical basis for spinal manipulation. In: Haldeman S, editor. Principles and practice of chiropractic. 3rd edition. New York: McGraw-Hill; 2005. p. 361–81.

16. Lederman E. The biomechanical response. Fundamentals of manual therapy: physiology, neurology and psychology. St Louis (MO): Churchill Livingstone; 1997. p. 23–37.

17. Bronfort G, Haas M, Evans RL, et al. Efficacy of spinal manipulation and mobilization for low back pain and neck pain: a systematic review and best evidence synthesis. Spine J 2004;4:335–56.

18. Threlkeld AJ. The effects of manual therapy on connective tissue. Phys Ther 1992;72:893–902.

19. Lederman E. Changes in tissue fluid dynamics. In: Lederman E, editor. Fundamentals of manual therapy: physiology, neurology and psychology. St Louis (MO): Churchill Livingstone; 1997. p. 39–54.

20. Gruenenfelder FI, Boos A, Mouwen M, et al. Evaluation of the anatomic effect of physical therapy exercises for mobilization of lumbar spinal nerves and the dura mater in dogs. Am J Vet Res 2006;67:1773–9.

21. Bergmann TF. High-velocity low-amplitude manipulative techniques. In: Haldeman S, editor. Principles and practice of chiropractic. 3rd edition. New York: McGraw-Hill; 2005. p. 755–66.

22. Cameron MH. Physical agents in rehabilitation. Philadelphia: W.B. Saunders Company; 1999.

23. Bolton PS, Budgell BS. Spinal manipulation and spinal mobilization influence different axial sensory beds. Med Hypotheses 2006;66:258–62.

24. Pickar JG. Neurophysiological effects of spinal manipulation. Spine J 2002;2:357–71.

25. Schmid A, Brunner F, Wright A, et al. Paradigm shift in manual therapy? Evidence for a central nervous system component in the response to passive cervical joint mobilisation. Man Ther 2008;13:387–96.

26. Hurwitz EL, Aker PD, Adams AH, et al. Manipulation and mobilization of the cervical spine. A systematic review of the literature. Spine (Phila Pa 1976) 1996;21:1746–59 [discussion: 1759–60].

27. Decoster LC, Cleland J, Altieri C, et al. The effects of hamstring stretching on range of motion: a systematic literature review. J Orthop Sports Phys Ther 2005;35:377–87.

28. Frick A. Fitness in motion: keeping your equine's zone at peak performance. Guilford (CT): The Lyons Press; 2007.

29. Light KE, Nuzik S, Personius W, et al. Low-load prolonged stretch vs. high-load brief stretch in treating knee contractures. Phys Ther 1984;64:330–3.

30. Taylor DC, Dalton JD Jr, Seaber AV, et al. Viscoelastic properties of muscle-tendon units. The biomechanical effects of stretching. Am J Sports Med 1990; 18:300–9.
31. Blignault K. Stretch exercises for your horse. London: J. A. Allen; 2003.
32. Giovagnoli G, Plebani G, Daubon JC. Withers height variations after muscle stretching in horses. In: Conference book The Race and Endurance horse, Proceedings of the Conference on Equine Sports Medicine and Science. Oslo, Norway, September 24–26, 2004. p. 172–6.
33. Rose NS, Northrop AJ, Brigden CV, et al. Effects of a stretching regime on stride length and range of motion in equine trot. Vet J 2009;181:53–5.
34. Bandy WD, Irion JM. The effect of time on static stretch on the flexibility of the hamstring muscles. Phys Ther 1994;74:845–50.
35. da Costa BR, Vieira ER. Stretching to reduce work-related musculoskeletal disorders: a systematic review. J Rehabil Med 2008;40:321–8.
36. Nansel DD, Waldorf T, Cooperstein R. Effect of cervical spinal adjustments on lumbar paraspinal muscle tone: evidence for facilitation of intersegmental tonic neck reflexes. J Manipulative Physiol Ther 1993;16:91–5.
37. Verschooten F. Osteopathy in locomotion problems of the horse: a critical evaluation. Vlaams Diergeneeskd Tijdschr 1992;61:116–20.
38. Bronfort G, Haas M, Evans R. The clinical effectiveness of spinal manipulation for musculoskeletal conditions. In: Haldeman S, editor. Principles and practice of chiropractic. 3rd edition. New York: McGraw-Hill; 2005. p. 147–66.
39. Herrod-Taylor EE. A technique for manipulation of the spine in horses. Vet Rec 1967;81:437–9.
40. Evrard P. Introduction aux techniques ostéopathiques struturelles appliquées au cheval. Thy-Le-Château (Belgium): Olivier éditeur; 2002.
41. Pusey A, Colles C, Brooks J. Osteopathic treatment of horses—a retrospective study. Br Osteopathic J 1995;16:30–2.
42. Haussler KK, Bertram JEA, Gellman K. In-vivo segmental kinematics of the thoracolumbar spinal region in horses and effects of chiropractic manipulations. Proc Amer Assoc Equine Pract 1999;45:327–9.
43. Haussler KK, Erb HN. Pressure algometry: objective assessment of back pain and effects of chiropractic treatment. Proc Amer Assoc Equine Pract 2003;49:66–70.
44. Sullivan KA, Hill AE, Haussler KK. The effects of chiropractic, massage and phenylbutazone on spinal mechanical nociceptive thresholds in horses without clinical signs. Equine Vet J 2008;40:14–20.
45. Wakeling JM, Barnett K, Price S, et al. Effects of manipulative therapy on the longissimus dorsi in the equine back. Equine Comp Exerc Physiol 2006;3:153–60.
46. Faber MJ, van Weeren PR, Schepers M, et al. Long-term follow-up of manipulative treatment in a horse with back problems. J Vet Med A Physiol Pathol Clin Med 2003;50:241–5.
47. Gomez Alvarez CB, L'Ami JJ, Moffat D, et al. Effect of chiropractic manipulations on the kinematics of back and limbs in horses with clinically diagnosed back problems. Equine Vet J 2008;40:153–9.
48. Chaitow L. Palpation skills. New York: Churchill Livingston; 1997.
49. Kessler RM, Hertling D. Assessment of musculoskeletal disorders. In: Hertling D, Kessler RM, editors. Management of common musculoskeletal disorders: physical therapy principles and methods. 2nd edition. Philadelphia: J.B. Lippincott; 1990. p. 68–71.

50. Haussler KK. Review of manual therapy techniques in equine practice. J Equine Vet Sci 2009;29:849–69.
51. Haussler KK. Chiropractic evaluation and management of musculoskeletal disorders. In: Ross MW, Dyson S, editors. Diagnosis and management of lameness in the horse. 2nd edition. St Louis (MO): Elsevier Saunders; 2011. p. 892–901.
52. Haussler KK. Equine chiropractic: general principles and clinical applications. Proc Amer Assoc Equine Pract 2000;46:84–93.
53. West DT, Mathews RS, Miller MR, et al. Effective management of spinal pain in one hundred seventy-seven patients evaluated for manipulation under anesthesia. J Manipulative Physiol Ther 1999;22:299–308.
54. Levine JM, Adam E, MacKay RJ, et al. Confirmed and presumptive cervical vertebral compressive myelopathy in older horses: a retrospective study (1992-2004). J Vet Intern Med 2007;21:812–9.
55. Rubinstein SM. Adverse events following chiropractic care for subjects with neck or low-back pain: do the benefits outweigh the risks? J Manipulative Physiol Ther 2008;31:461–4.
56. Stevinson C, Ernst E. Risks associated with spinal manipulation. Am J Med 2002; 112:566–71.
57. Senstad O, Leboeuf-Yde C, Borchgrevink C. Frequency and characteristics of side effects of spinal manipulative therapy. Spine 1997;22:435–40 [discussion: 440–1].
58. Rubinstein SM, Leboeuf-Yde C, Knol DL, et al. The benefits outweigh the risks for patients undergoing chiropractic care for neck pain: a prospective, multicenter, cohort study. J Manipulative Physiol Ther 2007;30:408–18.
59. Oliphant D. Safety of spinal manipulation in the treatment of lumbar disk herniations: a systematic review and risk assessment. J Manipulative Physiol Ther 2004; 27:197–210.
60. Dabbs V, Lauretti WJ. A risk assessment of cervical manipulation vs. NSAIDs for the treatment of neck pain. J Manipulative Physiol Ther 1995;18:530–6.

Kinesio Taping Fundamentals for the Equine Athlete

Sybille Molle, DVM, CERT, CKTIE

KEYWORDS

- Kinesio taping • Equine rehabilitation • Musculoskeletal diseases • Posture
- Complementary therapy

KEY POINTS

- Kinesio equine tape is lightweight, breathable, and allows full range of motion. It can be left on 24 hours a day for up to 5 days.
- The application of the tape on the skin can affect all of the layers of tissues and organs because they are all intimately interconnected.
- Kinesio taping application can relieve pain, increase range of motion, assist tissue recovery, optimize muscle function, and promote lymphatic flow.
- Kinesio taping assists rehabilitation of the horse in any phase; its main goal is to help the body's self-healing potential to bring tissues back to their homeostasis.

Absent a correct diagnosis, medicine is poison, surgery is trauma and alternative therapy is witchcraft.

—A. Kent Allen.

INTRODUCTION

Kinesio taping was first introduced in 1979 by Dr Kenzo Kase, a Japanese chiropractor and moxibustion practitioner (**Fig. 1**), as an efficient alternative to other wrapping or bandaging techniques already in use such as McConnell taping, compressive bandaging, and so on.

The idea underlying the invention of Kinesio Tex Tape was to have a tool working on the patients in between treatments. The consideration that all other types of bandages were in some ways restricting the range of motion and could not be worn longer than a few hours led Dr Kase to develop a particular type of elastic tape that could stay on for up to 5 days 24 hours per day.

Kinesio taping has been used for years, but it really broke out with 2008 Olympic Games when it had its first big media attention because it was used by many athletes.

The author has nothing to disclose.
Private Practice, Strada Fossaccio, 34, Viterbo 01100, Italy
E-mail address: sybille_molle@virgilio.it

Vet Clin Equine 32 (2016) 103–113
http://dx.doi.org/10.1016/j.cveq.2015.12.007
0749-0739/16/$ – see front matter © 2016 Elsevier Inc. All rights reserved.
vetequine.theclinics.com

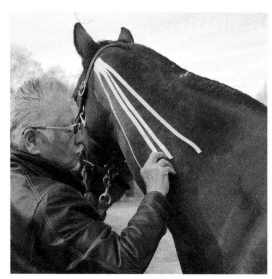

Fig. 1. Kenzo Kaze, the founder of Kinesio taping.

Since then, it has become usual to see it on athletes in almost all sports, although its main use remains in normal people's everyday life.

At the beginning of this century, the discovery of its potential use in animals and especially in equine athletes led many companies to develop equine taping as a very new and useful technique to be used in horses (**Fig. 2**).

Kinesio taping has been showing a great potential of application in almost all conditions that can be found in the equine athlete, from the competition ground to rehabilitation facilities. Especially in equine rehabilitation, it can be used to assess and treat muscular conditions, postural imbalances, and fascia restrictions; it has a great effect

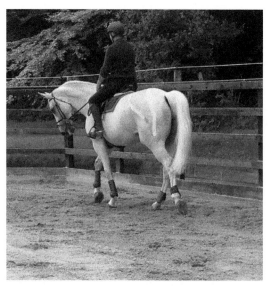

Fig. 2. Use of Kinesio taping in horses.

on tendon and ligament injuries and can also be used in lymphatic conditions. The taping assists the rehabilitation of the horse in any phase, because its main goal is to help the body's self-healing potential to bring tissues back to homeostasis.[1] It can be combined with other modalities or treatments, before or after the sessions, to prepare or complete the effect (**Fig. 3**).

It is important to keep in mind that Kinesio taping is not a substitute for veterinary care, its use needs to be approved by a clinician, and its application must be performed by trained professionals because improper use may be harmful.

MECHANISM OF ACTION
Characteristics of the Tape

The tape is produced with 100% cotton elastic fibers, which allows the skin to breathe and the tape to dry.[2] It stretches along its longitudinal axis only up to 130% to 140% of its resting length in a way that is similar to the flexibility of skin. The tints are all made of hypoallergenic dyes naturally derived from plant extracts; there is no difference in the physical characteristics of the tape depending on the dye used, but some chromotherapy effect is considered to be acting based on the color used for the treatment:

- Green: emotional calm, rebuild muscles, and help injuries;
- Yellow: mental alertness, optimism, aids digestion; and
- Brown: natural, earthy color.

The adhesive of Kinesio equine is 100% medical grade, acrylic, and heat activated; it is specifically designed to fit with the equine movement. The tape is not medicated and eventual feelings of warmth or cooling of the therapeutic zone are related to the direct effect on local circulation.

Embryology Concept

The application of the tape on the skin can affect all of the layers of tissues and organs because all stratums are intimately interconnected (**Fig. 4**). The relationship is even stronger for tissues that differentiate from the same layer (ie, epidermis and brain). The application of the tape on the skin affects 5 major physiologic systems differently:

- Skin: lifting effect with creation of space between superficial layers.
- Fascia: unwinding effect, redirection of movement.

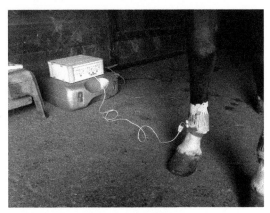

Fig. 3. Combined use of Kinesio taping and modalities.

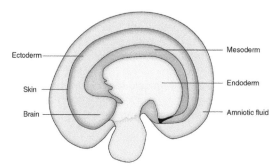

Fig. 4. Embryology concept. All layers are deeply interconnected.

- Muscle: optimization of function.
- Lymphatic: decongestion and fluid redirection.
- Joint: realignment effect through direct proprioceptive action on ligaments or indirect through muscle control.

Inflammation Concept

Inflammation is characterized by 5 fundamental elements: calor, rubor, tumor, dolor, and function lesa (ie, heat, redness, edema, pain, and loss of function). The Kinesio taping method aims to act on all of these components to reduce inflammation. The direct effect of the tape applied to the skin reduces heat, redness, and congestion through a direct action on the local circulation. The reduction of the edema and the decompressive action of this elastic bandage unloads the mechanoreceptors, thus promoting a pain-controlling effect. Finally, reduction of inflammation and the possibility to act on the range of motion through different techniques, which are discussed elsewhere in this article, helps to restore function.

Pressure Concept

Pain perception can be modulated by the tape's effect on the skin and fascia through the activation of the endogenous analgesic system[3,4] and the inhibitory pathways related to the pain-gate theory.[5] Either compressive or decompressive forces obtained by changing the tension of application can modulate pain. With compression, the mechanoreceptors will be stimulated, thereby activating the inhibitory pathways; in contrast, decompression unloads overworked receptors.

MUSCLE APPLICATIONS
Sensory–Motor Cortex Communication

Application of the tape on the skin stimulates sensory receptors, which produces an afferent message to the dorsal horn of the spinal cord and from there to the motor cortex through the ascending fibers where this is integrated with other proprioceptive stimuli to produce a motor response; in this way, the tape applied on the skin can affect the motor control of a muscle (**Fig. 5**). We can either rest an overused muscle through inhibition application or increase the motor awareness with facilitation.

Action of the Tape

Because of its intrinsic elasticity, after being applied the tape will recoil toward the starting point of application, and this directional pull travels through the tissues from the skin to the underlying muscles, thus stimulating the Golgi tendon organs and the muscle spindles. Proper location of the tape on specific anatomic landmarks, and the direction

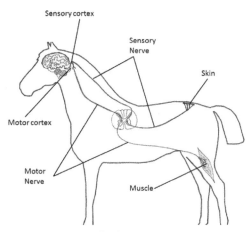

Fig. 5. Sensory–motor cortex communication.

and tension of application will achieve either an inhibiting or facilitating effect. More-over, depending on the condition diagnosed, the use of the tape will promote the resto-ration of the appropriate length of the muscle to produce the best contractile force (length–tension curve; **Fig. 6**), thus optimizing muscle function.

Use of Muscle Taping in Equine Rehabilitation

The effects of the tape on muscles are mainly to improve muscle balance, optimize the range of motion, relieve pain, and promote tissue recovery.[6] Application of the tape should be considered whenever there would be a primary muscle involvement, such as strains or tears, in case of metabolic conditions (ie, tying up), or neurologic pathologies with local muscle effects (ie, radial nerve paralysis). Moreover, muscle applications can be used when the participation of the muscles is needed to address or diagnose postural imbalances or gait abnormalities, to reeducate proper neuromotor control and to prevent injuries or repeat injuries in the rehabilitation process of many conditions (**Fig. 7**).

TENDONS AND LIGAMENTS
Corrective Techniques and Proprioceptive Awareness

Within the Kinesio taping method, different corrective techniques exist; one technique is designed for ligaments and tendons. The mechanism of action is based on the pro-prioceptive information given by the application of the tape to the skin in the area cor-responding with the tissue that needs treatment, the effect will be to support the ligament or tendon through the motor response elicited by the proprioceptive input.[7] The combination with techniques such as lymphatic or space correction will help to reduce the edema and to promote pain relief.

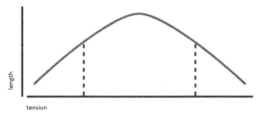

Fig. 6. Length–tension curve.

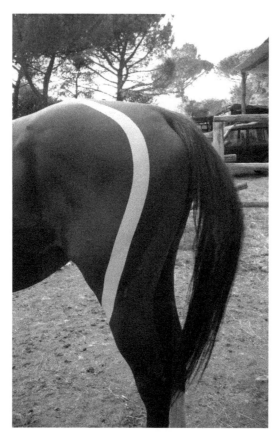

Fig. 7. Taping for biceps femoris facilitation.

Use of Ligament or Tendon Correction in Equine Rehabilitation

Depending on the stage of the injury or rehabilitation program, different options are possible. Most of the time, a combination of different applications is used. As a general indication, although the decision of the treatment protocol remains case dependent, the application of the tendon or ligament correction should be avoided in the early stages of inflammation or injury during which phase a lymphatic or space correction is more appropriate considering their effect on local circulation and pain. Once the inflammatory phase is achieved, the use of ligament or tendon correction (**Fig. 8**) is very useful to prevent overstretch of the tissue and to reeducate appropriate joint mobility; tendon correction can be combined with a muscle taping either in facilitation or inhibition depending on the stage of rehabilitation.

KINESIO TAPING AND FASCIA

The myofascial compartment is one of the actual rolling topics in both human and equine medicine and physical therapy. It is being demonstrated that especially superficial fascia is responsible for a majority of pathologic conditions in different areas of the body, and that it has the capacity to adapt to movement and to self-contract similarly to smooth muscles,[8,9] consequently influencing biomechanics. Many orthopedic

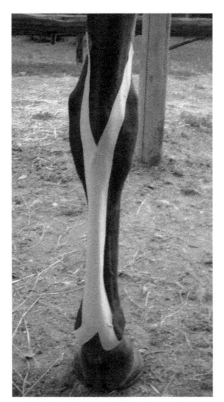

Fig. 8. Tendon correction.

conditions leave major gait or postural abnormalities, even after the primary problem is corrected, and it is considered that fascia is responsible for the maintenance of these anomalies.[10] This is why the treatment of fascia gains greater importance especially in the rehabilitation programs. The fascia is best treated manually through different techniques including myofascial release at first, but also osteopathy or chiropractic, the use of taping within fascia treatment is of great value[11] because it can either prepare very hard tissues for manipulation or continue the action of the manual therapy in between visits.

Use of Kinesio Taping in the Treatment of Fascia

The use of tape for fascial treatment falls into the corrective technique and is known as fascia correction. The aim of this therapeutic application is to release, unwind, and redirect the movement of the fascia in the physiologic direction and it is achieved by using the typical recoil of the tape thus creating micromovements in the underlying tissues that unbound the adhesions and act as a continuous micromassage. Unwinding the fascia allows the restoration of the mobility of the skin over the muscles or joints thus promoting the return to the appropriate range of motion of the area treated[12] (**Fig. 9**).

LYMPHATIC TAPING
Channeling Concept

The application of the tape to the skin, because of recoil, creates a form of wrinkles called convolutions, which may be immediately apparent or become visible later on

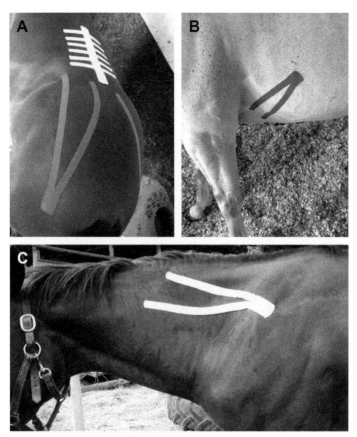

Fig. 9. Fascia correction. (*A*) thoracolumbar and gluteal fascia correction (*B*) fascia correction in girth area (*C*) fascia correction in the neck area.

depending on the elasticity of the underlying tissues; sometimes, they never come out because of the anatomic location (ie, horseback), but microconvolutions are present with movement. The convolutions create a pressure gradient by alternatively compressing and elevating the skin, thus promoting the fluid flow in the interstitial space with consequent improvement of circulation.[13,14]

Taping Application for Lymphatic Conditions

The evaluation of the lymphatic condition is crucial for the effectiveness of the lymphatic taping; the tape should never be applied to an area with active cellulitis and the use of lymphatic taping in patients with cardiac or kidney diseases has to be carefully monitored to avoid system overload. Lymphatic correction is very useful in a large number of circulatory conditions, from acute situations such as bruising or inflammatory edema to more chronic situations like lymphedema. The aim is to allow the fluid to move more freely in the interstitial space while directing it toward the closest healthy patent lymph nodes to be reabsorbed into the general circulation (**Fig. 10**).

USE OF KINESIO TAPING FOR JOINT DISEASES

Joint diseases are a common cause of poor performance in sport horses as described in a large number of papers present in scientific literature. There is a

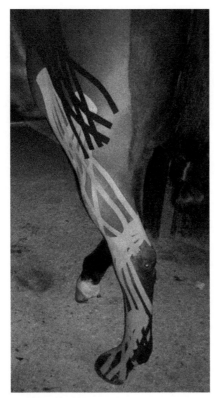

Fig. 10. Lymphatic taping of the hind limb.

wide range of causes to joint alterations such as diet, type of exercise, genetic predispositions, and so on. A highly contributing factor is malalignment in the joint motion causing overload in some areas of the cartilage or subchondral bone and inflammation of all the structures related to the joint such as capsule or ligaments. Kinesio taping applications can help in addressing the problem in 2 different ways:

- *Directly*, by acting on the ligaments that support the joint using a ligament correction thus giving proprioceptive feedback and consequent muscular action to correct the improper alignment[15]; and
- *Indirectly*, by acting on the muscles through facilitation and/or inhibition techniques thus rebalancing the muscular action and support in the joint area.[6]

A New Perspective: The Epidermis, Dermis, Fascia Taping

A newly introduced concept within the Kinesio taping method is called Epidermis, Dermis, Fascia.[16] Initially designed and tested in human neurologic conditions such as phantom sensations in amputated subjects, it was then brought into more wide range of use for many clinical conditions (ie, multiple sclerosis, local pain, and edema). Because of the very high sensitivity that horses showed to many taping applications, this technique is now starting to be used in the equine patients and showed very good results in the treatment of articular conditions (**Fig. 11**).

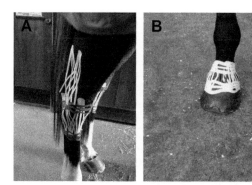

Fig. 11. Epidermis, dermis, fascia taping (*A*) hock (*B*) distal interphalangeal joint.

INDICATIONS FOR KINESIO TAPING TREATMENT

Kinesio taping can be used for a very large number of clinical conditions. It is considered that everything that can be treated with the hands can be treated with the tape. Potential applications include the following conditions:

- Tendon and ligament injuries;
- Muscle imbalances;
- Postural adjustments;
- Lymphatic and circulatory conditions;
- Neurologic pathologies;
- Pathologic movement patterns;
- Fascial adhesions;
- Scars; and
- Acute and chronic pain.

When using Kinesio taping applications, it must be kept in mind that there are some important contraindications, such as the use over active cellulitis, skin infection, open wounds, and malignancy sites. Taping should be used carefully in some clinical conditions such as kidney disease, congestive heart failure, and metabolic or endocrine disease.

FUTURE STUDIES

The effects of Kinesio taping application in various conditions are being largely investigated in human medicine and in the past years many scientific articles have been published and a huge amount of research is being performed as the medical community realized the need to have more answers regarding the mechanism of action and the potential applications in human medicine either to accelerate healing processes or to improve quality of life, especially in patients with cancer and neurologic conditions.[17] In veterinary medicine, the technique is very new and a few studies[18–20] have been already performed; further clinical research is needed to investigate the effects and the potentials of the use of Kinesio taping in equine rehabilitation and sports medicine.

REFERENCES

1. Kase K, Wallis J, Kase T. Clinical therapeutic applications of the Kinesio taping methods. Tokyo: Kinesio Taping Association; 2013.

2. Kase K, Molle S, Collins G. KTE1: fundamental concepts of the Kinesio taping method for horses. Albuquerque (NM): Kinesio Taping Association; 2014.
3. Watkins LR, Mayer DJ. Organization of endogenous opiate and nonopiate pain control systems. Science 1982;216(4551):1185–92.
4. Basbaum AL, Fields HL. Endogenous pain control systems: brainstem spinal pathways and endorphin circuitry. Annu Rev Neurosci 1984;7:309–38.
5. Melzack R, Wall PD. Pain mechanisms a new theory. Science 1965;150(3699): 971–9.
6. Cho HY, Kim EH, Kim J, et al. Kinesio taping improves pain, range of motion and proprioception in older patients with knee osteoarthritis: a randomized controlled trial. Am J Phys Med Rehabil 2015;94(3):192–200.
7. Kase K, Molle S, Collins G. KTE2: Kinesio taping equine concepts and corrective techniques. Albuquerque (NM): Kinesio Taping Association; 2014.
8. Tomasek JJ, Gabbiani G, Hinz B, et al. Myofibroblasts and mechanoregulation of connective tissue remodeling. Nat Rev Mol Cell Biol 2002;3(5):349–63.
9. Schleip R, Klingler W, Lehmann-Horn F. Fascia is able to contract in a smooth muscle-like manner and thereby influence musculoskeletal mechanics. In: Proceedings of the 5th world Congress of Biomechanics. Munich (Germany): Medimond; 2006. p. 51–4.
10. Guimberteau JC, Sentucq-Rigall J, Panconi B, et al. Introduction to the knowledge of subcutaneous sliding system in humans. Ann Chir Plast Esthet 2005; 50(1):19–34.
11. Wei-Ting W, Chang-Zern H, Li-Wei C. The Kinesio taping method for myofascial pain control [Review]. Evid Based Complement Alternat Med 2015;2015:950519.
12. Soo-Yong K, Min-Hyeok K, Ehi-Ryong K, et al. Effects of Kinesio taping on lumbopelvic-hip complex kinematics during forward bending. J Phys Ther Sci 2015;27:925–7.
13. Smith JY, Lee HR, Lee DC. The use of elastic adhesive tape to promote the lymphatic flow in the rabbit hind leg. Yonsei Med J 2003;44(6):1045–52.
14. Kase K. Illustrated Kinesio taping manual. 2nd edition. Tokyo: Kent-Kai; 1997.
15. Simon S, Garcia W, Docherty CL. The effect of Kinesio tape on force sense in people with functional ankle instability. Clin J Sport Med 2014;24(4):289–94.
16. Kase K, Molle S, Collins G. KTE3: Kinesio taping equine advanced and clinical concepts. Albuquerque (NM): Kinesio Taping Association; 2014.
17. Kara OK, Uysal SA, Turker D, et al. The effects of Kinesio taping on body functions and activity in unilateral spastic cerebral palsy: a single-blind randomized controlled trial. Dev Med Child Neurol 2015;57:81–8.
18. Molle S, Ruggeri D, D'Onofrio M. Use of Kinesio taping method in the treatment of sacro-iliac joint dysfunction in the horse: 7 cases. Short Communication, 7th IAVRPT Symposium. Vienna, August 15–18, 2012.
19. Clark L, Nankervis KJ. A pilot study investigating the effects of Kinesio taping on the gait characteristics of three horses. Gloucester (United Kingdom): The Equine Therapy Centre, Hartpury College; 2010.
20. Lima de Mattos LH, Miluzzi Yamada AL, Alves Rodrigues K et al. Application of Kinesio taping on postoperative equine stringhalt syndrome: case report. Poster Presentation, Brazilian Congress of Kinesio Taping. Brazil, 2013.

Principles and Application of Hydrotherapy for Equine Athletes

Melissa R. King, DVM, PhD

KEYWORDS

- Hydrotherapy • Underwater treadmill exercise • Buoyancy • Osmolality
- Hydrostatic pressure • Viscosity

KEY POINTS

- Exercising in water is an effective treatment option for managing musculoskeletal injuries.
- Hydrotherapy provides an effective medium for increasing joint mobility, enhancing muscle activation, improving postural control, and reducing inflammation.
- Various forms of hydrotherapy are frequently prescribed for rehabilitation of equine musculoskeletal injuries with the goal of improving the overall function of the affected limb and preventing further injuries.

INTRODUCTION

Aquatic rehabilitation has long been recognized as having beneficial effects in humans. Hydrotherapy is a commonly prescribed treatment option for managing primary musculoskeletal injuries and reducing or limiting harmful compensatory gait abnormalities in people.[1] Exercising in water provides an effective medium for increasing joint mobility, promoting normal motor patterns, increasing muscle activation, and reducing the incidence of secondary musculoskeletal injuries caused by primary joint pathology.[2] Humans with lower extremity osteoarthritis show a significant increase in limb-loading parameters, improved joint range of motion, and a significant reduction in the severity of balance deficits following aquatic exercise.[3] The enhancements in muscle strength and function associated with aquatic exercise also significantly improve proprioceptive deficits, poor motor control, and abnormal locomotor characteristics typically found in osteoarthritic adults.[4]

Author Declaration of Interests: No conflicts of interest have been declared.

Department of Clinical Sciences, College of Veterinary Medicine and Biomedical Sciences, Colorado State University, 300 west drake street, Fort Collins, CO 80526, USA

E-mail address: Melissa.king@colostate.edu

Vet Clin Equine 32 (2016) 115–126

http://dx.doi.org/10.1016/j.cveq.2015.12.008

0749-0739/16/$ – see front matter Published by Elsevier Inc.

vetequine.theclinics.com

PROPOSED MECHANISMS OF ACTION

Hydrotherapy interventions, such as underwater treadmill exercise and swimming, have been reported to reduce mechanical stresses applied to the limb, improve joint range of motion, decrease pain and inflammation, improve muscle strength and timing, and increase cardiovascular endurance.[5] The physical properties of water provide a medium where the mechanisms of increased buoyancy, hydrostatic pressure, and viscosity, along with the ability to alter temperature and osmolality, are applied in different combinations to play an important role in individualized musculoskeletal rehabilitation (**Fig. 1**). The increased resistance and buoyancy inherent in aquatic exercise increases joint stability and reduces weight-bearing stresses on muscles and joints.[6–8] Immersion of the distal limb causes circumferential compression, which increases proportionately with water depth. The increased extravascular hydrostatic pressure promotes circulation and reduces edema.[5] Hydrotherapy can also aid in decreasing pain through temperature effects. Immersion in warm water causes vasodilation, increased circulation, and decreased muscle spasms,[9] whereas cold water acts to reduce inflammation by restricting blood flow and reducing the accumulation of inflammatory mediators.[10] Aquatic conditions with higher solute concentrations provide an osmotic effect, which can ultimately reduce edema and decrease pain.[11] Hydrotherapy is a versatile treatment modality capable of producing a wide variety of therapeutic effects and therefore is considered an effective method for addressing sensory and motor disturbances associated with musculoskeletal injuries to achieve functional restoration of full athletic performance.[12]

Buoyancy

In the context of hydrotherapy, buoyancy is defined as a lifting force that acts to reduce axial loading of the joints by minimizing vertical ground reaction forces. Underwater force platform analysis of human subjects demonstrates a significant reduction

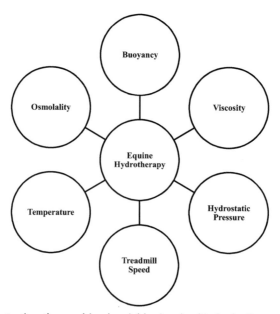

Fig. 1. Graph illustrating the combined variables involved in hydrotherapy.

in vertical ground reaction forces during walking,[3] which is inversely correlated with the depth of water immersion. Humans walking at a slow pace in water at the level of the manubrium have a 75% reduction in weight bearing, but only a 25% reduction in weight bearing when walking in water at level of the pelvis.[13] In horses, water at the level of the tuber coxae produces a 75% reduction in body weight, whereas water at elbow height has a 10% to 15% reduction in weight bearing.[14] Increased buoyancy reduces the effects of weight-bearing stress placed on joints and the surrounding soft tissue structures, which helps to reduce pain and inflammation associated with impact loading exercises. Underwater kinematic analysis in humans has also demonstrated that increased buoyancy improves joint range of motion. Humans with lower extremity osteoarthritis show increased limb flexion while walking in water compared with relatively decreased joint range of motion when walking on land.[15] The buoyancy effects of aquatic therapy can produce kinetic and kinematic effects that are directly applicable to the clinical management of musculoskeletal morbidities in horses.

Viscosity

The viscosity (fluid's resistance to flow) of water is about 12 times greater than that of air; therefore, the increased effort required to move through water causes increased muscle activation and improves muscle strength, motor control, and joint stability.[3] Electromyographic analysis during underwater exercise in human patients demonstrates increased activation of the agonist muscles during concentric contractions.[15] Increased agonist muscle activity is required to accelerate the limb in the direction of movement. However, during the same concentric contraction a reduced coactivation of the antagonist muscle group occurred.[15] Concentric muscle contractions during land locomotion cause the antagonist muscles to become activated to help decelerate the limb segments in preparation for foot contact. However, when exercising in water the increased resistance applied in the direction of motion requires minimal muscular braking of the limb segments.[15] Humans with knee osteoarthritis routinely demonstrate an inhibition of the quadriceps muscle group and a corresponding increase in the activity of the antagonist hamstring muscle group. The increased activation of the hamstring muscles is a normal compensatory mechanism that helps to stabilize the knee and to attenuate joint-loading forces during locomotion.[16] The increased resistance to limb movement provided by aquatic therapy reactivates the agonist muscles and reduces co-contraction of paired antagonist muscles, which enhances neuromuscular control and the coordination of muscle activity. These mechanisms are important contributors to the functional restoration of muscle function and motor control in the rehabilitation of various musculoskeletal injuries.

Hydrostatic Pressure

The immersion of the distal limb in water applies a circumferential compression of equal magnitude increasing extravascular hydrostatic pressure, which in turn promotes venous return and lymphatic drainage. The improved venous and lymphatic circulation reduces edema and decreases soft tissue swelling that ultimately increases joint range of motion and decreases pain.[5] Changes in hydrostatic pressure can also improve neuromuscular function by enhancing muscle spindle activity through the stimulation of skin surface sensory nerves and joint mechanoreceptors. These specialized receptors function as proprioceptors and as modifiers of muscle activity to increase joint stability and to protect joint structures from excessive or abnormal loading.[17] Reflex mechanisms mediated by joint receptors help to protect an injured joint from further damage via either inhibition or activation of muscular guarding in response to joint pain.[18] The joint mechanoreceptors also register mechanical deformation of the joint capsule and changes in intra-articular pressure during joint loading. The increase in intra-articular pressure associated with joint effusion and synovitis causes reflex afferent excitation of 1b interneurons located within the ventral horn of the spinal cord, which results in inhibition of the muscles that act on that joint.[19] Afferent excitation of joint mechanoreceptors induced by increased intra-articular pressure may be dampened by the effects of increased hydrostatic pressure when the limb is immersed in water.[5] The reduced inhibition of the spinal cord 1b interneurons causes increased activation of the alpha motor neurons, which produces increased muscle activation and tone. Reduced soft tissue swelling and joint effusion may further improve synaptic information from the joint mechanoreceptors and re-establish neuromuscular control critical for optimal joint motion and athletic activity.

Temperature

The thermodynamic properties of water provide markedly different therapeutic effects depending on temperature.

Cryotherapy

Cryotherapy is widely used in horses with the goal of decreasing acute soft tissue inflammation, pain, and swelling. The optimal therapeutic effects of cold hydrotherapy are generated through reducing tissue temperatures to 15°C to 10°C.[20] The application of cryotherapy produces peripheral vasoconstriction and decreased soft tissue perfusion (up to 80%), which can reduce edema formation and swelling at the site of tissue injury.[21] Reduced blood flow to the extremities also decreases tissue metabolism and provides an analgesic effect by decreasing nerve conduction velocity.[10] Local mechanisms of action include decreased tissue metabolism via reduced inflammatory mediator release, inhibition of degradative enzymatic activity, reduction of cellular oxygen demands, and decreased subsequent hypoxic injury.[22] Cold therapies can penetrate up to 1 to 4 cm in depth, which depends on local circulation and adipose tissue thickness.[23] Human studies have documented the analgesic benefits of cryotherapy with a 15- to 20-minute application providing pain relief for 1 to 2 hours.[24,25] In horses, a single report described the use of cryotherapy to treat lipopolysaccharide-induced synovitis, which concluded that twice-daily treatment for 2 hours was not effective for controlling inflammation.[26] However, ice water immersion for 30 minutes reduced the superficial and subcutaneous tissues in the distal limb to within optimal therapeutic range compared with cold pack application.[27] Although temperatures measured during cold pack application to the equine distal limb for 30 minutes did not fall within the optimal therapeutic range. Application of a compression boot with continuous circulating coolant applied to the distal forelimb of horses for 1 hour significantly reduced the Superficial digital flexor tendon (SDFT) core temperature to 10°C.[20] Similarly, a dry sleeve perfused cuff with continuous circulating coolant was as effective as ice-water immersion that included the hoof and distal limb in reducing hoof wall surface temperatures to less than 10°C during an 8-hour period.[28] In humans and dogs, circulating cryotherapy and intermittent compression provides a significant reduction in pain, swelling, lameness, and an increase in joint range of motion after orthopedic surgery.[29,30] The recent results of tissue cooling being as effective with circulating cryotherapy units compared with ice water immersion enhances efficacy and safety in the clinical application of cryotherapy. Further in vitro research has demonstrated that the viability of tenocytes exposed to cold treatment (10°C) for 1 hour did not significantly differ from those cells maintained at 37°C.[28] Cryotherapy research in horses has focused primarily on applications within the distal limbs and on inflammatory responses associated with laminitis.[31] The exact effect of cryotherapy on various equine musculoskeletal injuries has not been fully elucidated. Additional studies are needed to create evidence-based guidelines on the use of cryotherapy. These must address effective duration, frequency, temperature, and safety of application that will optimize outcomes after injury.

Thermotherapy

Thermotherapy often used in humans following the acute inflammatory phase is defined as an optimal therapeutic tissue temperature ranging from 40°C to 45°C.[27] Warm water immersion at 36°C causes vasodilation, which reduces peripheral vascular resistance and increases tissue perfusion.[9] Increased soft tissue perfusion may aid in dissipating inflammatory mediators associated with local inflammation and pain.[5] Water temperature during aquatic exercise may also play an important role in nociception by acting on local thermal receptors, and increasing the release of endogenous opioids.[32] Horses that stood in warm (38°C–40°C) spring water for 15 minutes demonstrated an increase in parasympathetic nervous system activity, indicating that immersion in warm spring water may have a relaxing effect that aids in decreasing pain, muscle spasms, and improves healing.[33] In humans, exercising in warm water has been shown to be an effective method for decreasing pain and enhancing joint range of motion. To date, there are no studies that demonstrate a clinical effectiveness for the use of warm water in the management of musculoskeletal disorders in horses. However, the physiologic effects of cold and warm water on vascular tone and tissue metabolism provide a useful tool to address the different inflammatory stages of musculoskeletal injury.

Osmolality

Exercising in water with higher solute concentrations has been reported to have anti-inflammatory, osmotic, and analgesic effects.[11] In humans, a 2-week course of daily exercise in mineral water demonstrated increased mechanical nociceptive thresholds (ie, reduced pain) over the medial aspect of osteoarthritic femorotibial joints.[34] Similarly, humans with fibromyalgia report significant improvements in pain scores lasting up to 3 months following exercise in a sulfur pool.[35] Horses diagnosed with distal limb injuries stood in hypertonic (20 g/L sodium chloride, 30 g/L magnesium sulfate) cold water baths (5°C–9°C) for 10 minutes, 3 days a week for 4 weeks (**Fig. 2**).[36] These horses demonstrated clinical and ultrasonographic healing of digital flexor tendon and suspensory ligament lesions.[36] Visual improvements in the degree of soft tissue swelling were also demonstrated within 8 days of the initiation of hypertonic cold water therapy.[36] In horses, tendonitis and desmitis monitored ultrasonographically demonstrated reduced peritendinous and periligamentous edema, decreased inflammatory infiltration, and improved collagen fiber alignment after the 4 weeks of hypertonic cold water therapy.[36] The added mineral components in water provide an increased osmotic effect, which reduces soft tissue inflammation and swelling, decreases pain, and ultimately improves joint range of motion. These osmotic effects can play an important role in managing soft tissue changes associated with musculoskeletal injury in horses.

EFFICACY OF HYDROTHERAPY

Although hydrotherapy is widely used in rehabilitation programs, there are few investigations into the benefits of this form of exercise for equine patients. Equine investigations involving hydrotherapy focus mainly on the horse's physiologic responses to exercising in water.[37–39] Swim training programs provide improvements in cardiovascular function, reductions in musculoskeletal injury (eg, tendonitis), and increases in fast-twitch, high-oxidative muscle fibers, which reflect improved aerobic

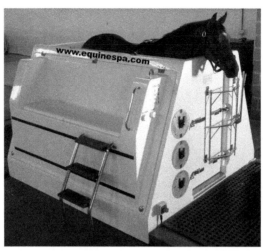

Fig. 2. Hypertonic cold water bath. (*Courtesy of* ECB Equine Spa, Sparta, NJ; with permission.)

capacity.[40,41] Fine-wire electromyography has been used to measure increased muscle activation of the thoracic limb musculature during pool swimming exercise, compared with overground walking.[42] More recently, changes in stride parameters have been assessed while horses walked in various depths of water.[43] Underwater treadmill exercise with water at the level of the ulna produced increased stride lengths and reduced stride frequencies, compared with walking in water at the level of the pastern joint.[43] A similar study assessed the influence of water depth on distal limb joint range of motion.[44] The varied depths of water (from <1 cm water height to the level of the stifle joint) significantly influenced the fetlock, carpal, and tarsal joint range of motion.[44] Results of this study demonstrate that water at varying depths promotes joint-specific increases in ranges of motion, therefore providing the ability to adapt therapeutic protocols to target certain joints. Changes in water depth also influence thoracolumbar lateral bending, pelvic flexion, and axial rotation. As water depth increases from hoof to shoulder level there is an increase in pelvic flexion and axial rotation but a decrease in lateral bending through the thoracolumbar region.[45] A study assessing the efficacy of underwater treadmill exercise to diminish the progression of experimentally induced carpal osteoarthritis was completed at the Colorado State University, Equine Orthopedic Research Center.[46] This project was established to provide an objective assessment of the pathologic characteristics associated with osteoarthritis and the potential clinical and disease-modifying effects allied with aquatic therapy. Underwater treadmill exercise was able to re-establish baseline levels of passive carpal flexion, returning the carpal joint to full range of motion. In addition, horses exercised in the underwater treadmill demonstrated evenly distributed thoracic limb axial loading, symmetric timing of select thoracic limb musculature, and significant improvements in static balance control under various stance conditions. The improvement in clinical signs of osteoarthritis in the aquatic therapy group was further supported by evidence of disease-modifying effects at the histologic level. Underwater treadmill exercise reduced joint capsule fibrosis and decreased the degree of inflammatory infiltrate present in the synovial membrane. Results from this study provide an objective assessment of the pathologic characteristics associated with osteoarthritis and the potential clinical and disease-modifying effects allied with underwater treadmill exercise, which is fundamental to providing evidence-based support for equine aquatic therapy.[46] However, additional studies focusing on developing methodology and the exact effect of hydrotherapy on more frequently treated musculoskeletal injuries are required.

HYDROTHERAPY VARIABLES

Equine hydrotherapy primarily involves the use of underwater treadmills (above ground or in ground units), swimming pools (circular or straight), aquawalkers, and standing salt water spas or whirlpools. The in-ground underwater treadmills by design have the capacity to hold a greater amount of water and thus provide more buoyancy in comparison with the above-ground underwater treadmill units. The above-ground underwater treadmill units are able to change the depth of water between each patient, allowing for targeted rehabilitation protocols designed to improve joint range of motion (**Fig. 3**). Both underwater treadmill units can come installed with hydrojets creating additional turbulent fluid flow, which increases the resistance of limb movement through the water-enhancing muscle strength and timing. In addition, underwater treadmill units have the ability to vary the treadmill speed, water temperature, and solute concentration. Horses frequently require a period of 3 to 5 days to become acclimated and trained to exercise in the underwater treadmill units.

The aquawalkers are mechanical walkers fitted within a circular pool that contains a consistent depth of water. The diameter of the aquawalker dictates how many horses can be exercised at a time; most systems are able to exercise six to eight horses simultaneously. Horses are not completely buoyant and are separated from each other by dividers creating an individual "pen" for each horse. The depth of the water is dictated by the system design; some have just a shallow trough with water maintained no higher than the fetlock joint, whereas others maintain the water height at the level of the stifle joint. The speed of system is controlled; however, unlike the underwater treadmills the horse may not walk at the consistent speed set by the unit. Some horses choose to slow down and then rush forward was the divider approaches them from behind only to slow down again once they catch up to the divider in front of them. Similar to the underwater treadmill units the aquawalkers are able to vary the water temperature and solute concentration.

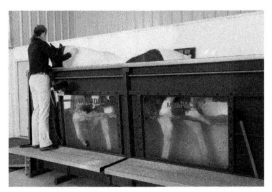

Fig. 3. Underwater treadmill. (*Courtesy of* Hudson Aquatic Systems, LLC, Angola, IN; with permission.)

Swimming horses typically takes place in linear or circular shaped pools with ramps installed for ease of entry and exit. Equine pools should be designed so that handlers on each side of the horse's head can walk alongside during each exercise session. To ensure complete buoyancy the water depth should be more than 12 feet deep. Linear pools may decrease cardiorespiratory stress as the horse is allowed to recover on exiting while being walked back to the entry point.[47] Conversely, continuous lap swimming in circular pools does not allow for cardiorespiratory recovery until completion of the exercise session. Horses are not natural swimmers and often use their thoracic limbs to maintain balance while the pelvic limbs are primarily used for propulsion. The explosive nature of the pelvic limb propulsion often results in extreme ranges of motion through the hip, stifle, and hock joints. In addition, on entry into the water horses often adopt a posture that results in cervical, thoracolumbar, and pelvic extension. In the authors opinion swimming horses with thoracolumbar, sacroiliac, hip, stifle, and hock injuries should be approached with caution.

PRECAUTIONS

Swimming horses with respiratory disease should be avoided because the increase in hydrostatic pressure influences lung volume, preventing adequate ventilation.[38] Aquatic therapy should also be avoided if the horse has any of the following conditions:

- Unhealed surgical incisions
- Open, infected, draining wounds
- Upper pelvic limb lameness
- Thoracolumbar pain/injury
- Acute joint inflammation
- Acute myositis
- Elevated temperature
- Fearful or panicky animal
- Cardiovascular compromise

TREATMENT PROTOCOL CONSIDERATIONS

The development of hydrotherapy rehabilitation protocols should be designed to meet the needs of each individual patient following a complete assessment and understanding of the desired long-term goals for athletic performance. Not only should the injury and physical conditions be considered, but understanding the temperament, behavioral response to water exposure, and previous history of aquatic therapy are crucial to developing a solid therapeutic plan. The development and progression of a hydrotherapy program should involve three main components: (1) intensity, (2) duration, and (3) frequency of applied therapy. The depth of water, turbulence, and speed of walking can influence intensity of exercise in the underwater treadmill. It is difficult to control intensity while swimming, and most horses are allowed to select a self-determined pace. However, some linear pools can provide a higher intensity work load by having horses swim against a current. The initial duration of treatment is greatly influenced by the nature of the injury, body condition, fitness level preinjury and postinjury, and the presence of muscle weakness and/or atrophy. Initially horses may only be able to exercise in the underwater treadmill for 5 minutes in the first week of therapy. The goal is to be able to increase the duration of walking by 5-minute increments weekly until 20 minutes is reached. Similarly, swimming sessions may involve only being able to swim one or two laps initially (5–8 minutes), working up to swimming (continuously for circular pool) for a total of 9 to 12 laps. The frequency of treatment is often dictated by response of the horse to the rehabilitation program. Typically the more intensive the exercise program the faster the return to function as long as the injury is not overloaded and is given time to adapt and strengthen.[48] Most underwater treadmill protocols are designed for daily aquatic therapy, 5 days a week. Swimming protocols range from three times a week, to 15-minutes sessions three times a week combined with 5-minute sessions twice a week. It is critical to remember when progressing within a rehabilitation program that only one aspect of the protocol should be changed at a time. If intensity and duration are changed simultaneously, then these changes may be too much too soon.

MONITORING PROCEDURES

Monitoring recovery heart rates is a useful tool in recognizing when a horse can progress in their rehabilitation program. Heart rates and recovery rates can be monitored before, during, and immediately following exercise to quantify the level of intensity. The heart rate during aquatic therapy should not exceed 200 beats per minute and the time required for the heart rate to decrease to 60 beats per minute should be less than 10 minutes. Rehabilitation therapeutic protocols should not increase in intensity if target heart rate is exceeded or if there is an extended recovery period.

The ability to quantitatively assess injury regression is crucial to monitoring the efficacy of therapeutic interventions. Evidence-based practice requires the use of valid, reliable, and sensitive tools to monitor treatment effectiveness. Pressure algometry, goniometry, and limb circumference are reliable and objective methods of determining pain, joint range of motion, swelling, and muscle mass and are often used to assess articular responses to physical therapy.[49] Horses should be evaluated daily before each aquatic therapy session for any palpable musculoskeletal defects in the affected limb and for any alterations in the degree of lameness. If appropriate, ultrasonography should be repeated at monthly intervals to assist in adjusting the rehabilitation protocols.

SUMMARY

Hydrotherapy incorporates several different mechanisms of action, all of which have particular benefit in the management of equine musculoskeletal disorders. The current human and veterinary literature suggests that aquatic therapy has beneficial effects on multiple musculoskeletal morbidities, such as pain reduction and increased joint range of motion. Well-designed, controlled, clinical trials using hydrotherapy are needed in horses to determine dosages effects (eg, water level, duration, and speed) and to assess clinical changes in soft tissue swelling, joint stability, and motor control patterns associated with adaptive and maladaptive compensatory gait alterations. The diverse physical characteristics of hydrotherapy provide unique approaches to individualized rehabilitation of musculoskeletal issues in horses.

REFERENCES

1. Hurley M. The effects of joint damage on muscle function, proprioception and rehabilitation. Man Ther 1997;2(1):11–7.
2. Prins J, Cutner D. Aquatic therapy in the rehabilitation of athletic injuries. Clin Sports Med 1999;18:447–61.
3. Miyoshi T, Shirota T, Yamamoto S-I, et al. Effect of the walking speed to the lower limb joint angular displacements, joint moments and ground reaction forces during walking in water. Disabil Rehabil 2004;26(12):724–32.

4. Messier S, Royer T, Craven T, et al. Long-term exercise and its effect on balance in older, osteoarthritic adults: results from the fitness, arthritis, and seniors trial (FAST). J Am Geriatr Soc 2000;48:131–8.

5. Kamioka H, Tsutanji K, Okuizumi H, et al. Effectiveness of aquatic exercise and balneotherapy: a summary of systematic reviews based on randomized controlled trials of water immersion therapies. J Epidemiol 2010;20:2–12.

6. Evans B, Cureton K, Purvis J. Metabolic and circulatory responses to walking and jogging in water. Res Q 1978;49:442–9.

7. Nakazawa K, Yano H, Miyashita M. Ground reaction forces during walking in water. Medicine and Science in Aquatic Sports 1994;39:28–34.

8. Hinman R, Heywood S, Day A. Aquatic physical therapy for hip and knee osteoarthritis: results of a single-blind randomized controlled trial. Phys Ther 2007;87: 32–43.

9. Yamazaki F, Endo Y, Torii R, et al. Continuous monitoring of change in hemodilution during water immersion in humans: effect of water temperature. Aviat Space Environ Med 2000;71:632–9.

10. Buchner H, Schildboeck U. Physiotherapy applied to the horse: a review. Equine Vet J 2006;38:574–80.

11. Bender T, Karagulle Z, Balint GP, et al. Hydrotherapy, balneotherapy, and spa treatment in pain management. Rheumatol Int 2005;25:220–4.

12. Masumoto K, Takasugi S, Hotto N, et al. Electromyographic analysis on walking in water in healthy humans. J Physiol Anthropol Appl Human Sci 2004;23(4):119–27.

13. Harrison R, Hilman M, Bulstrode S. Loading of the lower limb when walking partially immersed: implications for clinical practice. Physiotherapy 1992;78: 164–6.

14. McClintock SA, Hutchins DR, Brownlow MA. Determination of weight reduction in horses in floatation tanks. Equine Vet J 1987;19:70–1.

15. Poyhonen T, Keskinen K, Kyrolainen H, et al. Neuromuscular function during therapeutic knee exercise underwater and on dry land. Arch Phys Med Rehabil 2001; 82:1446–52.

16. Dixon J, Howe T. Quadriceps force generation in patients with osteoarthritis of the knee and asymptomatic participants during patellar tendon reflex reactions: an exploratory cross-sectional study. BMC Musculoskelet Disord 2005; 6:1–6.

17. Salo P. The role of joint innervation in the pathogenesis of arthritis. Can J Surg 1999;42:91–100.

18. Iles J, Stokes M, Young A. Reflex actions of knee joint afferents during contraction of the human quadriceps. Clin Physiol 1990;10:489–500.

19. Hopkins J, Ingersoll C, Krause B, et al. Effect of knee joint effusion on quadriceps and soleus motoneuron pool excitability. Med Sci Sports Exerc 2001;33: 123–6.

20. Petrov R, MacDonald MH, Tesch AM, et al. Influence of topically applied cold treatment on core temperature and cell viability in equine superficial digital flexor tendons. Am J Vet Res 2003;64:835–44.

21. Worster AA, Gaughan EM, Hoskinson JJ, et al. Effects of external thermal manipulation on laminar temperature and perfusion scintigraphy of the equine digit. N Z Vet J 2000;48:111–6.

22. Algafly AA, George KP. The effect of cryotherapy on nerve conduction velocity, pain threshold and pain tolerance. Br J Sports Med 2007;41:365–9 [discussion: 369].

23. Brosseau L, Rahman P, Toupin-April K, et al. A systematic critical appraisal for non-pharmacological management of osteoarthritis using the appraisal of guidelines research and evaluation II instrument. PLoS One 2014;9:e82986.

24. Sanchez-Inchausti G, Vaquero-Martin J, Vidal-Fernandez C. Effect of arthroscopy and continuous cryotherapy on the intra-articular temperature of the knee. Arthroscopy 2005;21:552–6.

25. Guillot X, Tordi N, Mourot L, et al. Cryotherapy in inflammatory rheumatic diseases: a systematic review. Expert Rev Clin Immunol 2013;10:281–94.

26. Hassan K, MacDonald M, Petrov R, et al. Investigation of the effects of local cryotherapy on intra-articular temperature and experimentally induced synovitis in horses. Proceedings 21st Annual Meeting Association of Equine Sports Medicine. Sacramento, CA, September 20–22, 2001. p. 70–2.

27. Kaneps AJ. Tissue temperature response to hot and cold therapy in the metacarpal region of a horse. Proceedings American Association of Equine Practitioners 2000;46:208–13.

28. van Eps AW, Orsini JA. A comparison of seven methods of continuous therapeutic cooling of the equine digit. Equine Vet J 2016;48(1):120–4.

29. Drygas KA, McClure SR, Goring RL, et al. Effect of cold compression therapy on postoperative pain, swelling, range of motion, and lameness after tibial plateau leveling osteotomy in dogs. J Am Vet Med Assoc 2011;238:1284–91.

30. Bleakley CM, Costello JT. Do thermal agents affect range of movement and mechanical properties in soft tissues? A systematic review. Arch Phys Med Rehabil 2012;94:149–63.

31. Pollitt CC, van Eps AW. Prolonged, continuous distal limb cryotherapy in the horse. Equine Vet J 2004;36:216–20.

32. Coruzzi P, Ravanetti C, Musiari L, et al. Circulating opioid peptides during water immersion in normal man. Clin Sci (Lond) 1988;74:133–6.

33. Kato T, Ohmura H, Hiraga A, et al. Changes in heart rate variability in horses during immersion in warm springwater. Am J Vet Res 2003;64:1482–5.

34. Yurtkuran M, Yurtkuran M, Alp A, et al. Balneotherapy and tap water therapy in the treatment of knee osteoarthritis. Rheumatol Int 2006;27:19–27.

35. McVeigh J, McGaughey H, Hall M, et al. The effectiveness of hydrotherapy in the management of fibromyalgia syndrome: a systematic review. Rheumatol Int 2008; 29:119–30.

36. Hunt E. Response of twenty-seven horses with lower leg injuries to cold spa bath hydrotherapy. J Equine Vet Sci 2001;21:188–93.

37. Voss B, Mohr E, Krzywanek H. Effects of aqua-treadmill exercise on selected blood parameters and on heart-rate variability of horses. J Vet Med A Physiol Pathol Clin Med 2002;49:137–43.

38. Hobo S, Yosjida K, Yoshihara T. Characteristics of respiratory function during swimming exercise in thoroughbreds. J Vet Med Sci 1998;60:687–9.

39. Nankervis KJ, Williams RJ. Heart rate responses during acclimation of horses to water treadmill exercise. Equine Vet J Suppl 2006;(36):110–2.

40. Misumi K, Sakamoto H, Shimizu R. Changes in skeletal muscle composition in response to swimming training for young horses. J Vet Med Sci 1995;57: 959–61.

41. Misumi K, Sakamoto H, Shimizu R. The validity of swimming training for two-year-old thoroughbreds. J Vet Med Sci 1994;56:217–22.

42. Tokuriki M, Ohtsuki R, Kai M, et al. EMG activity of the muscles of the neck and forelimbs during different forms of locomotion. Equine Vet J Suppl 1999;(30): 231–4.

43. Scott R, Nankervis K, Stringer C, et al. The effect of water height on stride frequency, stride length and heart rate during water treadmill exercise. Equine Vet J Suppl 2010;(38):662–4.

44. Mendez-Angulo JL, Firshman AM, Groschen DM, et al. Effect of water depth on amount of flexion and extension of joints of the distal aspects of the limbs in healthy horses walking on an underwater treadmill. Am J Vet Res 2013;74: 557–66.

45. Mooij MJW, Jans W, den Heijer GJL, et al. Biomechanical responses of the back of riding horses to water treadmill exercise. Vet J 2013;198(Suppl 1):e120–3.

46. King M, Haussler K, Kawcak C, et al. Effect of underwater treadmill exercise on postural sway in horses with experimentally induced carpal osteoarthritis. Am J Vet Res 2013;74:971–82.

47. Bromiley MW. Equine injury, therapy and rehabilitation. 3rd edition. Ames (IA): Blackwell Publishing; 2007.

48. McGowan CM, Stubbs NC, Jull GA. Equine physiotherapy: a comparative view of the science underlying the profession. Equine Vet J 2007;39:90–4.

49. Gajdosik R, Bohannon R. Clinical measurement of range of motion. Phys Ther 1987;67:1867–72.

Electrophysical Therapies for the Equine Athlete

Carrie Schlachter, VMD*, Courtney Lewis, DVM

KEYWORDS

- Equine athlete • Electrophysical therapies • Rehabilitation • Treatment

KEY POINTS

- Electrophysical therapies are useful tools for therapy if used at the appropriate time and in the appropriate method.
- Some methods may be harmful to tissues during certain phases of healing.
- There is currently a lack of research in horses to support or reject the use of most of these modalities.

 Video content accompanies this article at http://www.vetequine.theclinics.com

INTRODUCTION

Rehabilitation is defined as restoring or bringing an animal to a condition of health or useful and constructive activity. A good rehabilitation program takes into account the possible causes for the injury. Although the specifics of this process can be difficult, the concepts are straightforward. Once the underlying cause of the injury is determined, a veterinarian can construct an appropriate rehabilitation plan and use the available electrophysical therapies to their greatest effect.

The when, how, and for how long of the electrophysical therapies can be simplified by understanding the goals and physical attributes of the modalities and the healing stages of the injured tissue. Most significant injuries have a 30-day inflammatory period, a variable filling-in phase (2–6 months), and then a hugely variable remodeling period (6 months to 2 years). Treating the horse correctly for the type and location of injury, and the stage of rehabilitation of the tissue, helps ensure full rehabilitation success.

From a functional perspective, the goals reflect the healing stages of the tissue. The first goal is to remove pain (inflammatory period). The second is to restore, maintain, or improve range of motion (controlled walking exercise, bodywork, other therapies). The third goal is to restore or improve strength (increased exercise,

Circle Oak Equine Sports Medicine, Petaluma, CA, USA
* Corresponding author.
E-mail address: carrieschlachter@gmail.com

Vet Clin Equine 32 (2016) 127–147
http://dx.doi.org/10.1016/j.cveq.2015.12.011
0749-0739/16/$ – see front matter

targeted rehabilitation techniques) in the injury and in the overall fitness level of the horse.

This article discusses when and how to use the most common electrophysical therapies in horses including transcutaneous electrical nerve stimulation (TENS), neuromuscular electrical stimulation (NMES), functional electric stimulation (FES), pulsed electromagnetic field therapy (PEMF), therapeutic ultrasound, laser therapy, shockwave therapy, and vibration therapy.

TRANSCUTANEOUS ELECTRICAL NERVE STIMULATION
Origin

The use of electricity for pain relief dates back to a story of an ancient Greek that stepped on an electric fish and noted a significant improvement in his own pain. This led to the development of the "electreat," a machine that was used through the early nineteenth century that used electricity to treat all manner of ailments. In the early 1960s the first portable TENS unit was developed and marketed for in-home pain relief.

Mechanism of Action

Electrostimulation provides pain relief primarily via segmental inhibition through pain gating mechanisms[1] (**Fig. 1**). This relies on activation of larger diameter fibers in peripheral nerves, which in turn helps block nociceptive activity in smaller afferents. Secondarily electric stimulation of peripheral nerves can stimulate a central release of endogenous opiate-like substances, which can have a descending inhibitory effect on pain.[2]

Treatment Protocols

Treatment parameters are based on electrical stimulation in the low-frequency range (<250 Hz) using appropriate pulse durations and intensities to activate the desired nerves. Large-diameter sensory nerves are activated first because of their proximity to the skin surface. Secondarily motor nerves are activated, then nociceptor nerves are affected via the pain gating mechanisms.[1]

Potential Complications

The contacts can cause skin irritation if left on for too long, so care should be taken to inspect the area of treatment regularly for evidence of irritation. Otherwise the modality has minimal complications when used properly.

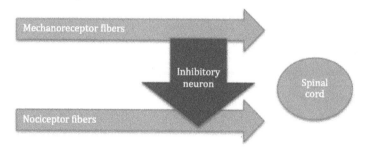

Fig. 1. Gate control theory. Mechanoreceptors can override the nociceptor pain response via presynaptic inhibition.

Indications for Use

- Electrical stimulation for pain modulation (**Table 1**)
- Acute pain associated with surgery or trauma
- Chronic musculoskeletal pain
- Muscle stimulation through the alpha motor nerve
- Stimulation of de-enervated muscles
- Iontophoresis
- Edema reduction
- Wound healing

Contraindications for Use

- Cardiac issues
- Pregnancy
- Do not use over or through the thoracic cavity
- Fevers or infection

Current Research

There is limited current research into the use of TENS therapy (**Fig. 2**) in horses. There seems to be some hope for using percutaneous electrical nerve stimulation to ameliorate the symptoms of trigeminally induced head shaking.[3] There is an abundant amount of research to support the use of TENS in humans for a variety of painful conditions.[4] A large portion of the recommendations for equine use is assumed from the human literature. Johnson's[4] book on TENS is a good source for the usefulness of TENS therapy in humans.

Table 1
TENS therapy summarized

TENS Therapy	Sensory TENS	Motor TENS	Noxious TENS
Also called	High-rate TENS	Low-rate or acupuncture-like TENS	Point stimulation
Use in	Any painful condition	Subacute pain or trigger point therapy	—
Avoid in	—	Acute conditions	—
Mechanism of action	Spinal gate mechanism	Descending mechanisms via endogenous opiate release	Central biasing mechanism
Efficacy	Quick relief; short lasting	Longer to effect; longer lasting	—
Nerves targeted	A-beta; large diameter	A-delta; fast pain	C-fiber
Amplitude	Submotor stimulation	Muscle contraction	As high as tolerable
Phase duration	<100 μs	200–300 μs	10–20 ms
Pulse rate	60–120 pps	2–4 pps	2–4 or 100–150 pps
Mode	Continuous/modulation	Continuous mode	—
Length of treatment	20–30 min or continuous	20–30 min	30 s/point; 8–10 points/session
Frequency of treatment	Continuously or intermittently throughout day	Intermittently throughout day	Intermittently throughout day

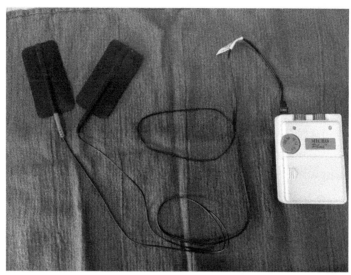

Fig. 2. TENS therapy device. (*Courtesy of* BioMedical Life Systems, Vista, CA; with permission.)

NEUROMUSCULAR ELECTRICAL STIMULATION
Origin

Generated from TENS, the goal of NMES is to achieve full contraction of a much larger muscle belly. The goal of FES is to mimic the pattern of intact nerves. The most commercially available neuromuscular stimulation unit manufactured for horses is the FES unit. NMES was first used in the rehabilitation of patients with spinal cord injury to generate muscle movement.[5] It has been used to prevent atrophy of de-enervated muscles and for a large range of nerve and muscle conditions to decrease pain or atrophy and improve function. The FES unit (**Fig. 3**, Video 1) has been adapted to provide pain relief and support for the equine athlete in training.

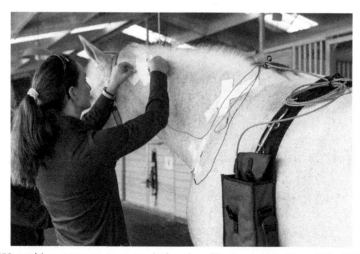

Fig. 3. FES machine set up to treat cervical region. (Equinew, LLC, Rivers Falls, WI.)

Mechanism of Action

Using the same electrical stimulation as the TENS unit the NMES machines use a longer pulse duration (width; 200–600 μs), variable amplitude needed to achieve muscle contraction, and a frequency of more than 50 Hz.

Treatment Protocols

The treatment goal is to achieve muscle contraction; therefore, proper placement of the electrodes and increasing the amplitude to effect is an effective way of constructing a treatment plan. The intensity should be what the animal can tolerate; the number of repetitions should start low (8–15 contractions per session) and increase to more than 3 to 5 weeks with one to five sessions per week depending on the treatment goal and injury.[5]

Potential Complications

Some horses are intolerant of the procedure. The same skin irritation can occur as with the TENS unit but less commonly because the treatment length is usually shorter.

Indications for Use

- Electrical stimulation for pain modulation (**Table 2**)
  - Acute pain associated with surgery or trauma
  - Chronic musculoskeletal pain
- Muscle stimulation through the alpha motor nerve
- Stimulation of de-enervated muscles
- Removal of edema

Contraindications for Use

- Cardiac issues
- Pregnancy
- Do not use over or through the thoracic cavity
- Fevers or infection

Current Research

Similar to the TENS research most research into neuromuscular electrical stimulation has been in humans. In horses FES (**Table 3**) has been shown to improve epaxial muscular contraction over time and to decrease muscle spasm.[6] There is minimal research apart from case studies and anecdotal evidence.

The human research has been wide ranging. In humans FES has been shown to help improve reaching and grasping functions,[7] and to reverse muscle atrophy in de-enervated muscle tissue.[8] Contrary to many claims there is also research showing that a good physical therapy program is effective with or without the addition of NMES for patellar femoral pain syndrome.[9]

ELECTROMAGNETIC ENERGY: PULSED ELECTROMAGNETIC FIELD THERAPY
Origin

The ancient Greek *magnes lithos* meaning, "stone from Magnesia," is the origin of the word "magnet." There is a larger percentage of the mineral magnetite in the rocks in the area of Magnesia. Magnetic stones were advocated to be therapeutic in ancient Chinese texts. Electrical generation of a magnetic wave was first proved in the time of Albert Einstein.[10] Modern electromagnetic field therapy started in 1971 when Friedenberg and coworkers[11] described the healing success of direct current

Table 2
TENS/NMES treatment parameters

Nerve Type	Characteristics	Examples	Phase Duration	Amplitude	Frequency
Aα	Motor fibers Diameter 13–20 μm Speed 80–120 ms⁻¹	Muscle spindle cells (primary) Golgi tendon organs Mechanoreceptors	250 μs	Sufficient to produce mm contractions	>50 pps
Aβ	Sensory fibers Low threshold Diameter 6–12 μm Speed 35–75 ms⁻¹	Mechanoreceptors Proprioceptors Muscle spindle cells (secondary)	<150 μs	Submotor	60–120 pps
Aδ	Sensory fibers High threshold Diameter 1–5 μm Speed 5–35 ms⁻¹	Mechanoreceptors Cold sensitive Nociceptors	200–300 μs	Strong muscle contractions	<10 pps
C	Sensory fibers Diameter <1.5 μm Speed <2 ms⁻¹	Nociceptors Mechanoreceptors Cold and heat sensitive	>300 ms	Pain response	<20 pps OR >100 pps
Muscle membrane	Stimulation of de-enervated muscle	—	n/a; direct current	n/a; direct current	≤5 mA
Sympathetic fibers	Microcurrent	—	Variable	Subsensory	Variable

Table 3
FES treatment protocols

Clinical Condition	Treatment Frequency	Length of Treatment
Thoracic/lumbar/sacral pain	2 within 28 h 3 within 3 wk 6 within 1 y	Variable; response to treatment
Kissing spine	2 within 48 h 3 within 3 wk 12 within 1 y	Variable; response to treatment
Muscle atrophy	2 within 48 h 3 within 3 wk 6 within 1 y	Until return to full function
Limb edema	2 within 48 h 3 within 3 wk 6 within 1 y	Until resolution of edema
Tendonopathy	2 within 48 h 3 within 3 wk 4–12 within 1 y	One year
Suspensory desmopathy	2 within 48 h 3 within 3 wk 4–12 within 1 y	One year or more

Data from Schils S. Equinew user manual (manual that came with FES machine). 2014.

delivered to a nonunion fracture. To be less invasive Bassett and coworkers[12] at Columbia University in the mid-1970s developed a protocol using low-frequency electromagnetic signals. Goodman and coworkers[13] also showed that there were changes occurring at the cellular level, but that these were not happening until 45 minutes of exposure to the waves.

Mechanism of Action

The therapeutic generation of local heat by high-frequency electromagnetic waves is called diathermy. The waves are generated as an electrical current is driven through a coiled wire. The magnetic field creates small currents inside the tissues. The greatest heating occurs in tissue with low impedance, such as muscles. Pulsed diathermy can raise temperatures of deeper tissues by 3°C to 4°C.[14] PEMF is a lower frequency and is derived from this heat-generating therapy (**Fig. 4**). Short wave diathermy can be adjusted to a low frequency (less than 600 pps) and short phase duration (65 s). This magnetic field results in currents within the tissues but no heating inside the tissues.

In the equine world there are several therapeutic options available for PEMF therapy. There are blankets and wraps with coils and energy-generating battery units built into them.[15] There are small coil systems[16] and large coil systems,[17] which produce the magnetic field in different sizes and strengths.

Treatment Protocols

The treatment protocols vary significantly in the literature and seem to be specific to the type and manufacturer of the machine used. They are based on the frequency of the pulses and the treatment time.

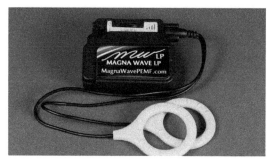

Fig. 4. Small PEMF machine. (*Courtesy of* Magna Wave PEMF, Louisville, KY; with permission.)

Potential Complications

There are minimal documented side effects from PEMF treatments.

Indications for Use

- Stimulate bone healing
- Increase blood flow in superficial and deep tissues
- Decrease pain and muscle spasm

Contraindications for Use

- Application over any implants
- Pregnancy
- Open wounds
- Cancer
- Infection
- Acute inflammation and joint effusion

Current Research

The strongest evidence for efficacy with PEMF lies with nonunion or slow to heal fractures (**Table 4**). There does not seem to be significant evidence to support soft tissue uses of PEMF in the horse or in humans.

Table 4 depicts the wide range of treatment parameters that have been researched in other species each of which has shown to have a positive effect on bone healing. However, in the 1980s in horses there was a study that showed no improvement in healing of osteotomies in groups treated with electromagnetic devices compared with control animals.[18]

Table 4 Treatment parameters for PEMF for bone healing			
	Frequency	Treatment Time	Length of Treatment
Bone healing in dogs[19]	1.5 Hz	1 h/d	8 wk
Delayed union[20]	15 Hz	3 h/d	—
Nonunion fracture[21]	7.5 Hz	8 h/d	30 d
Decreased pain postfracture	50 Hz	30 min/d	—

THERAPEUTIC ULTRASOUND
Origin

In the early twentieth century, following the tragic sinking of the Titanic, research began on the use of sound waves to identify objects. During the early phases, it was found to have detrimental effects on marine life, which led to its use in live tissues as a medical therapy. The first recorded use was in 1938 on a human suffering from sciatica.[22]

Mechanism of Action

Unlike diagnostic ultrasound, therapeutic ultrasound (**Fig. 5**) is designed specifically to have a biologic effect on the tissues. The ultrasound uses cyclic vibration frequencies of 1 to 3 MHz, and the mechanical energy produced makes for a wave of acoustic energy, which is inaudible to the human ear. This energy travels through tissues and is absorbed by the deep tissues via molecular vibration, without altering the temperature of the skin surface.[5]

- Good penetration while maintaining tissue selectivity
- Increases in temperature, which provides cellular energy
- Increased cellular metabolism
- Increased oxygen demand
- Causes vasodilation
- Allows inflammatory components to infiltrate the region
- Mast cells become activated and degranulate
- Triggers the arachidonic acid cascade developing a proinflammatory state[23]

Used during the proliferative phase of healing, therapeutic ultrasound can upregulate fibroblastic activity and increase protein and collagen synthesis via release of growth factors.[24]

In the remodeling phase of tendon and ligament healing, ultrasound can increase the tensile strength of collagen, improving the fiber pattern and orientation as it assists

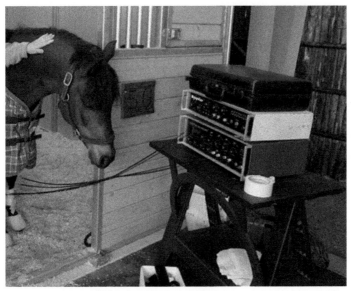

Fig. 5. Therapeutic ultrasound machine (DynaPacific Dynatronics Livermore Operation, CL, USA) in use on a bilateral deep digital flexor desmotomy.

in the transition from type 3 to type 1 collagen.[25] Therapeutic ultrasound frequencies are well absorbed from high-protein tissues, and minimally absorbed by tissues high in water content.

Cartilage and bone, although high in protein, reflect the ultrasound waves, so this therapy has no effect on these tissues.[26] Therapeutic ultrasound also has an analgesic effect likely via decreased local nerve conduction and the release of endorphins and serotonin.

There are also nonthermal effects of therapeutic ultrasound. This is via the cavitation that occurs from mechanical vibration energy that forms tiny gas bubbles that improve the acoustic streaming, therefore altering cellular diffusion and permeability. Sodium and calcium ion transport channels are most affected altering the membrane potential and cellular secretions.[27]

Therapeutic ultrasound is used in two different modes: pulsed and continuous. The pulsed mode provides nonthermal effects, such as cavitation and mechanical effects, whereas the continuous mode provides the thermal effects on the tissue.[28] Therapeutic ultrasound does not have a cumulative effect in treatment, meaning the tissue temperatures do not remain elevated for longer than the treatment itself (**Fig. 6**). A 1° increase in temperature triggers metabolic activity, 2° to 3° with decrease muscle spasms and increase blood flow, and 4° with change the viscoelastic properties of collagen.[5] The specific settings depend on the machine, but often treatments are started on a daily basis for up to 7 to 10 days then decreased to a few days per week until the desired effect is noted.

Potential Complications

There is a narrow window of temperature range, which can make use challenging and potentially risky. The ideal temperature for use is 40°C (104°F), but above 45°C (113°F) can cause tissue damage. The machines require maintenance and calibration to maintain appropriate temperatures. The ultrasound does not work through air, and therefore requires a clean patient, copious gel, and good transducer contact. Clipping the hair further improves the contact.[29]

Indications for Use

- Tendon and ligament: minimizes contraction with healing
- Fascial planes
- Joint capsule: improves range of motion
- Scar tissue: softens scar tissue
- Osteophytes/enthesiophytes: decreases pain; however, no effect on bone itself
- Muscle spasms: slows gamma fiber transmission
- Wounds: increases protein synthesis in fibroblasts (use 2 weeks postinjury)

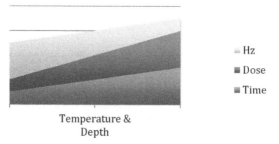

Temperature &
Depth

Fig. 6. Temperature versus depth chart for therapeutic ultrasound.

- Edema: reduces tissue edema[22]
- Nerve injuries: remyelination and regeneration of damaged axons[30]

Contraindications for Use

- Ophthalmic use: poor vascularization of lens causes intolerance to heat
- Pregnant mares: specifically over reproductive regions
- Cardiac: potential for electrical disruption
- Growth plates: potential for developmental abnormalities
- Fractures: may delay healing process
- Hindered sensation, such as nerve blocked locations
- Vascular insufficiency
- Thrombophlebitis/clotting dysfunction: potential for emboli
- Infection/cellulitis: potential for spread of infection via vasodilation
- Malignancy: potential for spread
- Immediately after exercise: tissues already at high temperature[22]

Current Research

A recent study on the thermal effects of ultrasound treated both the superficial and deep digital flexor tendons with a 3.3-MHz continuous ultrasound for 10 minutes at an intensity of 1.0 W/cm^2. This led to an approximate increase in temperature of 3°F to 7°F in the flexor tendon tissue. However, at the same settings of 3.3 MHz and 1.0 W/cm^2, there is no change in temperature detected in the epaxial muscles along the spine.[31]

In canines, a study looked at Achilles tendon injuries and found that those dogs treated with therapeutic ultrasound (0.5 W/cm^2) had improved tendon healing and their return to soundness was more rapid compared with those without therapeutic ultrasound.[32]

Therapeutic ultrasound has also been tested in the treatment of induced septic arthritis in donkeys, and those treated with ultrasound therapy had less changes to the joint capsule, synovium, and articular cartilage.[33]

EXTRACORPOREAL SHOCKWAVE THERAPY
Origin

Shockwave (extracorporeal shockwave therapy [ESWT]) has been used in medicine to break up ureteral stones in humans, but was not used in equine orthopedics until 1996, when a German veterinarian used it to treat suspensory desmitis.[34] At the time, the machines were very large and general anesthesia was required for equine patients.

Mechanism of Action

Shockwave (**Fig. 7**) uses pressure waves that increase as they travel through tissues. The pressure change leads to cavitation, and the formation and collapse of tiny gas

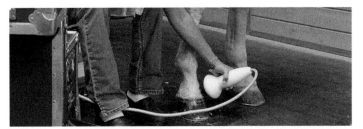

Fig. 7. Shockwave therapy being applied to medial distal interphalangeal joint collateral ligament.

bubbles, which leads to microtrauma of the tissues. This microtrauma is beneficial to the injured tissue in that it leads to neovascularization and therefore increased blood flow to the area. The increased blood blow allows for introduction of inflammatory cells and nutrients. Shockwave also has analgesic effects, which peak approximately 48 hours after treatment, this should be taken into consideration because this has the potential to mask the patient's pain level, which can be risky in the rehabilitating horse.[35]

Treatment Protocols

- Focal energy used (probe type) (**Table 5**)
- Number of pulses effect on tissues
- Upper limit where unwanted tissue damage can occur
- There is not a set range for these limits because they depend on
  - Patient's size
  - Location of the affected tissue
  - Individual machine

Shockwave is a therapy that uses the three-dimensional conformation of a patient and therefore the administrator must work from all angles on the affected area. Protocols for use generally require three to six treatments at 2- to 3-week intervals. Too frequent of use does not allow the body to react and initiate healing from the microtrauma that is produced.

- Good tissue contact is required, which may mean clipping hair, cleaning the area, and lots of ultrasound gel
- Shockwaves do not penetrate the hoof wall, sole, through a cast, or through an air interface

Table 5
Standard treatment protocols for ESWT

Location	# of Pulses	Energy Flux	Results
Fourth metatarsal bone stress fracture/exostosis	2000	.15 m/mm²	Increased exostosis
Tendon/ligament injury	600	.14 m/mm²	Increased Glycosaminoglycans Increase protein synthesis
Forelimb proximal suspensory desmitis	2000	.15 m/mm²	Increased intracellular matrix
Superficial digital flexor tendonitis	—	—	Faster healing Increased vascularization
Osteoarthritis of hock joints	2000	.89 m/mm²	Decreased protein in synovial fluid Improved lameness
Navicular syndrome (through frog between heel bulbs)	1000/1000	.89 m/mm²	56% improved one lameness grade
Collateral ligament of distal interphalangeal joint	—	—	No significant improvement compared with rest/controlled exercise
Back pain (bone sclerosis)	50 pulses/cm²	.15 m/mm²	—
Back pain (muscular)	100 pulses, trigger points	.15 m/mm²	—

- There seems to be better efficacy for shockwave therapy on the front limbs compared with the hind limbs[36–38]
- Shockwaves generally penetrate a maximum of 50 to 110 mm, thus making deeper structures, such as the sacroiliac joint, out of their treatment range[39]
- Shockwave treatment of collateral ligaments of the distal interphalangeal joints is not positively correlated with outcomes[40]

Potential Complications

It is rare, but with overuse, tissues can become overheated. Swelling has been seen at the affected site posttreatment. There is potential for development of white hairs over the treated area. Treatment on bone has the potential to exacerbate microfracture damage with excessive numbers of pulses used. Shockwave does not function through an air interface, such as the thoracic cavity, and reflects, which has the potential to lead to hemorrhage. Good tissue contact is required, which means clipping hair, cleaning the region, and copious amounts of gel.

Indications for Use

- Tendon/ligament injuries or desmitis/tendonitis: rapid healing, improved fiber pattern, matures collagen fibers
- Bone (including stress fractures, exostoses, osteoarthritis): osteogenic stimulation and remodeling
- Nonhealing fractures: improve callus formation
- Periostitis
- Back pain
- Frog: can penetrate hoof through frog if treating distal phalanx

Contraindications for Use

- Young, growing animals: can lead to premature closure of physes

Current Research

Most of the current research on ESWT entails experimentally induced tendon and ligament injuries, such as forelimb and hindlimb suspensory ligament desmitis via the introduction of collagenases into the tissues. The studies on forelimbs and hindlimbs showed the limbs treated with ESWT had more collagen fibril formation, increased growth factors (transforming growth factor-β), and increased proteoglycan deposition. Ultrasonographically, the lesions showed improved healing with less hypoechogenicity and smaller lesion size.[41,42] Shockwave therapy also was seen to decrease the degree of lameness seen in these horses. This is likely caused by a period of analgesia that occurs approximately 4 days post-ESWT treatment. Because of this analgesic effect of shock wave therapy, both the federation equestre internationale and Racing Jurisdiction of the United States have implemented regulations regarding specific withdrawal times before competition. There has also been research on the effects of ESWT on bone pathology. A study using arthroscopically induced osteoarthritis of the middle carpal joint in horses found that those treated with ESWT had no evidence of adverse effects and lameness was visibly improved. Shockwave did not show direct evidence of benefits to the synovial fluid or tissue or the associated articular cartilage of the arthritic joint.[34,43]

LASER THERAPY
Origin

Laser therapy has been in use for more than 30 years, and has really taken off in the veterinary field for small and large animals in the last 10 years. Laser has similar benefits as acupuncture, but without the invasiveness of the needles, and is often used on similar trigger points.[44]

Mechanism of Action

There are four classes of lasers, with the class IV laser (**Fig. 8**) being the most common choice for equine practice. These low-level lasers work in a range less than 500 mW, and the wavelengths vary from 540 nm to 1060 nm. Laser therapy, similarly to therapeutic ultrasound and shockwave, has anti-inflammatory and analgesic effects.

- Stimulates cellular metabolism
- Direct activation of mitochondrial calcium channels
- Upregulation of ATP production and synthesis
- Increases fibroblastic activity[45]
- Increased cellular division, fibroblast migration, and production of cellular matrix[45]

More specifically, it has been shown that prostaglandin E_2, tumor necrosis factor-α, interleukin-1β, plasminogen activator, and cyclooxygenase-1 and -2 are all manipulated with the use of laser therapy, producing a decrease in inflammation.[46] The anti-inflammatory effect is via stimulation of prostaglandins leading to vasodilation.[47]

Laser therapy is beneficial on wounds and tendon and ligament injuries, because it increases cellular proliferation and collagen synthesis leading to more rapid healing of the damaged tissue. Laser therapy works synergistically with platelet-rich plasma treatments to increase recovery time in tendon and ligament injuries, such as tenosynovitis and synovitis. Not only has laser therapy been shown to accelerate healing, but it can also be used to maintain optimum performance, and prevent recurrence of injury.[15]

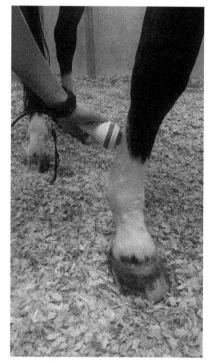

Fig. 8. Laser therapy for a superficial digital flexor injury.

The effects of laser therapy on bone are partially unknown; however, there have been several studies showing benefits in dental procedures in humans, leading to bone repair and regeneration.[45]

Treatment Protocols

Proper use of low-level laser therapy depends on the machine used. Considerations are wavelength, pulse frequency, and time of application. If not used properly the tissues can overheat so it is important to follow product labels and directions. Laser can be used on a daily, weekly, or monthly basis for treatment and/or prevention. Often for injuries treatments begin daily then decrease over time depending on response to treatment.[48] A study on the use of laser therapy on wound healing treated the wound every other day for 80 days with great results. Treatment time varies based on location and purpose of treatment and wavelength and power of the machine. Generally the treatment time varies from 5 to 30 minutes.[49]

Potential Complications

Other than the previously mentioned contraindications, potential concerns with laser therapy include overheating the tissues with overuse or incorrect use. Care should be taken to follow the appropriate machine indications and protocols. Another concern with the use of laser therapy is damage to both the patient's and the administrator's cornea. Protective eyewear should be worn when performing laser therapy, and eye shields should be placed on the horse if the treatment is in the head or neck region.

Indications for Use

- Performance maintenance
- Prevention of injury recurrence
- Synergistic with stem cell and platelet-rich plasma treatment
- Tendon and ligament injury
- Chronic joint disease
- Synovitis
- Osteoarthritis
- Back pain/injury
- Wound healing
- Pain relief
- Neurologic injuries
- Alternative to acupuncture/acupressure

Contraindications for Use

- Pregnant mares (unknown effect)
- Young, growing animals (unknown effect on physes)
- Malignancy
- Hematologic disorders
- Febrile patients
- Ocular use

Current Research

There is growing research on the effects of laser therapy on wound healing. There is conflicting evidence regarding the effect of laser on second-intent wound healing, because some studies have shown no significant differences in epithelialization or wound contraction.[50] Another study looking at two horses with septic wounds found that laser therapy stimulated fibroblastic formation and collagen synthesis.[51] In studies in species other than equine, histologic responses to low-level laser therapy have indicated a reduction in inflammation, reduction in edema, and increased collagen synthesis.[52] Further research on the efficacy of laser therapy on wound treatment is needed because of the varied results.

Low-level laser therapy is regularly used as a treatment modality for tendon and ligament damage. Minimal research has been done in equines in terms of effects on tendon and ligaments and joints and cartilage. A study done in rodents with collagenase-induced Achilles tendonitis showed reduction in matrix metalloproteases and improvement in the mechanical properties of the tendon.[46] Chemically induced osteoarthritis in rabbits treated with laser therapy indicated cartilage regeneration and chondrocyte replacement.[53] Both of these studies provide promising evidence that similar effects may occur in our equine patients.

VIBRATION THERAPY
Origin

Vibration plates (**Fig. 9**) were first developed for humans in the 1990s for treatment of osteoporosis. The plates were first developed for astronauts as a way to prevent osteoporosis and muscle wasting in the absence of gravity.

Mechanism of Action

Vibration plates provide mechanical energy in the vertical and/or horizontal direction, and the amplitude of the motion and speed of acceleration determine the ultimate magnitude of the vibration produced.[54] Vertical vibration more closely mimics the natural movement of the horse. Vibration plates are thought to improve circulation of the cardiovascular and lymphatic systems, via continuous involuntary muscle contractions (30–50 per second). Benefits of improving circulation include enhanced oxygenation of tissues, removal of toxic and metabolic waste, and introduction of cells as part of the inflammatory cascade.[55] Vibration plates also promote joint stability to some degree in that they directly stimulate and strengthen the associated muscles,

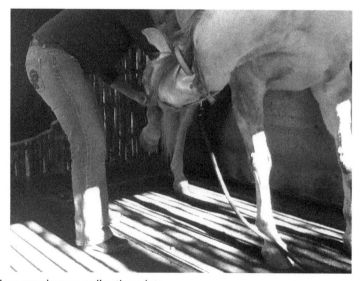

Fig. 9. Core exercises on a vibration plate.

such as in the human knee or equine stifle joint.[56] In humans, vibration plates have been used to assist in counteracting osteoporosis; however, results in horses have shown minimal to no osteoblastic activity.[57] Vibration plates also provide general feelings of well-being in that it has been shown to stimulate production of the neurotransmitter serotonin and decrease serum cortisol with low-intensity whole-body vibration.[57,58] Moderate to high intensity vibration behaves like extensive exercise, however, and increases creatinine kinase levels indicating muscle breakdown and elevated lactate levels caused by anaerobic metabolism.[59]

Treatment Protocols

Little research has been done on specific treatment protocols for the use of the various types of whole-body vibration plates. Anecdotally, they have been used on a daily basis in healthy animals with no ill effects. Sessions generally last 10 to 15 minutes, but should be modified based on the specific brand recommendations. It is suspected that pulsed treatment as opposed to continued vibration may have better osteogenic stimulation. In humans, frequencies in the range of 25 to 45 Hz led to improved muscle strength and an increase in muscle size.[54]

Potential Complications

The potential effects of whole-body vibration on a patient with any form of internal fixation are unknown and therefore should be avoided until further research has been conducted. Not all horses tolerate the vibration plate and, therefore, do not make good candidates for its use.

Indications for Use

- Tendon and ligament injuries
- Maintenance of fitness
- To promote blood flow
- Postoperative strength training (depending on surgery)

Contraindications for Use

- Acute fractures

Current Research

A 2013 study measured general clinical parameters in seven horses following 10 minutes of whole-body vibration exercise at a frequency of 25 to 21 Hz. The study found no measurable ill effects or signs of discomfort from the horses, in that their serum cortisol levels and creatinine kinase levels were significantly lowered following the treatment. No other clinical parameters were changed following the use of the vibration plate, including bone markers, suggesting there are no osteoblastic effects of vibration in horses.[57] A 2009 study in humans, however, showed significant osteogenesis and increased fluid flow through the extracellular spaces in bone and lacunae as a result of the loading forces from the vibration plate.[54] The same paper also showed a noticeable increase in testosterone levels, and this particular hormone is known to promote bone mineral density in humans. Similarly, growth hormone levels also increase with exercise and are suspected to also be elevated with vibration plate activation subsequently promoting osteogenesis.[54]

SUMMARY

Electrophysical therapies is an evolving field of rehabilitation that is growing faster than the scientific community can keep up (**Table 6**). These machines are manufactured by

Table 6
Summary of modalities

Appropriate Use of Modality During Healing Phases							
	TENS	NMES	PEMF	EWST	Laser	Therapeutic US	Vibration Therapy
Inflammatory	x	—	—	x	x	x	—
Filling in	x	x	—	x	x	x	x
Remodeling	x	x	x	x	—	—	x

Appropriate Use of Modalities for Specific Conditions							
Condition/Therapy	TENS	NMES/FES	PEMF	Therapeutic US	ESWT	Laser	Vibration Therapy
Arthritis	x	x	x	x	X	x	x
Back soreness	x	x	x	x	X	x	x
Cellulitis	x	x	—	—	—	x	—
Colic recovery	x	x	x	x	X	x	—
Hoof injuries	—	—	—	—	x(frog)	—	—
Acute laminitis	—	—	—	—	—	—	—
Chronic laminitis	—	—	—	—	—	—	—
Tendon and ligament injury	x	x	x	x	x	x	x
Muscle injury	x	x	x	x	—	x	x
Muscle soreness	x	x	x	x	x	x	x
Neurologic disease	x	x	—	—	—	x	—
Postsurgery recovery	x	—	—	x	—	x	—
Scar tissue/adhesions	x	x	x	x	x	x	—
Wounds	x	—	—	X (2 wk post)	x	x	—
Skin infections	x	—	—	—	—	—	—

many different companies in different places with a huge variation on quality and little to no safety oversight. Minimal peer-reviewed scientific studies are available; therefore, anecdotal evidence and case studies make up most of their claims of efficacy. The Internet is accessible to the horse owner, so it is easy to get a new technology out to the market. It seems proving the efficacy of the modality can be as simple as one good review by an Olympic champion on social media. This is not an ideal situation, because the veterinary community is falling behind the curve of knowledge. This article is not an exhaustive list of the electrophysical therapies available for equine rehabilitation today (an ever growing and expanding field). Future editions of this article may list some very different topics. It is hoped that time and more peer-reviewed research will provide more realistic expectations of treatment outcomes to discuss with our owners.

SUPPLEMENTARY DATA

Supplementary data related to this article can be found at http://dx.doi.org/10.1016/j.cveq.2015.12.011.

REFERENCES

1. Melzack R, Wall PD. Pain mechanisms: a new theory. Science 1965;150(3699): 971–9.

2. Walsh DM, Lowe AS, McCormack K, et al. Transcutaneous electrical nerve stimulation: effect on peripheral nerve conduction, mechanical pain threshold, and tactile threshold in humans. Arch Phys Med Rehabil 1998;79(9):1051–8.
3. Roberts VL, Patel NK, Tremaine WH. Neuromodulation using percutaneous electrical nerve stimulation for the management of trigeminal-mediated headshaking: a safe procedure resulting in medium-term remission in five of seven horses. Equine Vet J 2016;48:201–4.
4. Johnson M. Transcutaneous electrical nerve stimulation: review of effectiveness. Nurs Stand 2014;28(40):44–53.
5. Denegar CR, Saliba E, Saliba S. Therapeutic modalities for musculoskeletal injuries. 3rd edition. Champaign, IL: Human Kinetics Publishers; 1988.
6. Schils S. Functional electrical stimulation for equine epaxial muscles: retrospective study of 241 cases. Equine Comp Exerc Physiol 2014;10(2):89–97.
7. Thrasher TA, Zivanovic V, McIlroy W, et al. Rehabilitation of reaching and grasping function in severe hemiplegic patients using functional electrical stimulation therapy. Neurorehabil Neural Repair 2008;22(6):706–14.
8. Mushahwar VK, Jacobs PL, Normann RA, et al. New functional electrical stimulation approaches to standing and walking. J Neural Eng 2007;4(3):S181–97.
9. Bily W, Trimmel L, Mödlin M, et al. Training program and additional electric muscle stimulation for patellofemoral pain syndrome: a pilot study. Arch Phys Med Rehabil 2008;89(7):1230–6.
10. Encyclopedia Britannica.
11. Friedenberg ZB, Harlow MC, Brighton CT. Healing of nonunion of the medial malleolus by means of direct current: a case report. J Trauma 1971;11(10):883–5.
12. Bassett CA, Pawluk RJ, Pilla AA. Augmentation of bone repair by inductively coupled electromagnetic fields. Science 1974;184(4136):575–7.
13. Goodman R, Bassett CA, Henderson AS. Pulsing electromagnetic fields induce cellular transcription. Science 1983;220(4603):1283–5.
14. Draper DO, Knight K, Fujiwara T, et al. Temperature change in human muscle during and after pulsed short-wave diathermy. J Orthop Sports Phys Ther 1999; 29(1):13–8 [discussion: 19–22].
15. Respond Systems, I. Available at: http://www.respondsystems.com.
16. Magnafix. Available at: http://www.wehealanimals.com/Donlan/.
17. Magnawave. Available at: http://www.magnawavepemf.com.
18. Sanders-Shamis M, Bramlage LR, Weisbrode SE, et al. A preliminary investigation of the effect of selected electromagnetic field devices on healing of cannon bone osteotomies in horses. Equine Vet J 1989;21(3):201–5.
19. Machen MS, Tis JE, Inoue N, et al. The effect of low intensity pulsed ultrasound on regenerate bone in a less-than-rigid biomechanical environment. Biomed Mater Eng 2002;12(3):239–47.
20. Ibiwoye MO, Powell KA, Grabiner MD, et al. Bone mass is preserved in a critical-sized osteotomy by low energy pulsed electromagnetic fields as quantitated by in vivo micro-computed tomography. J Orthop Res 2004;22(5):1086–93.
21. Chen LP, Han ZB, Yang XZ. The effects of frequency of mechanical vibration on experimental fracture healing. Zhonghua Wai Ke Za Zhi 1994;32(4):217–9 [in Chinese].
22. Porter M. Therapeutic ultrasound, in the Horse. 1998.
23. Fyfe MC, Chahl LA. Mast cell degranulation and increased vascular permeability induced by 'therapeutic' ultrasound in the rat ankle joint. Br J Exp Pathol 1984; 65(6):671–6.

24. Vasquez B, Navarrete J, Farfán E, et al. Effect of pulsed and continuous therapeutic ultrasound on healthy skeletal muscle in rats. Int J Clin Exp Pathol 2014; 7(2):779–83.

25. Enwemeka CS, Rodriguez O, Mendosa S. The biomechanical effects of low-intensity ultrasound on healing tendons. Ultrasound Med Biol 1990;16(8): 801–7.

26. Lin Gelbmam, B., CVTP, ESMT, CCRP., Therapeutic Ultrasound.

27. EQ Ultrasound. Stable cavitation and acoustical streaming physiological effects. Available at: http://www.equltrasound.com/.

28. ter Haar G. Therapeutic applications of ultrasound. Prog Biophys Mol Biol 2007; 93(1–3):111–29.

29. Oke S. Therapeutic ultrasound settings for horses. The Horse; 2013.

30. Mourad PD, Lazar DA, Curra FP, et al. Ultrasound accelerates functional recovery after peripheral nerve damage. Neurosurgery 2001;48(5):1136–40 [discussion: 1140–1].

31. Montgomery L, Elliott SB, Adair HS. Muscle and tendon heating rates with therapeutic ultrasound in horses. Vet Surg 2013;42(3):243–9.

32. Saini NS, Roy KS, Bansal PS, et al. A preliminary study on the effect of ultrasound therapy on the healing of surgically severed Achilles tendons in five dogs. J Vet Med A Physiol Pathol Clin Med 2002;49(6):321–8.

33. Singh KI, Sobti VK, Roy KS. Gross and histomorphological effects of therapeutic ultrasound (1 Watt/Cm2) in experimental acute traumatic arthritis in donkeys. J Equine Vet Sci 1997;17(3):150–5.

34. Scott R, McClure D. Extracorporeal shock wave therapy in horses: what we know. 2003.

35. Loving N, Kent A, editors. Extracorporeal shock wave therapy: this noninvasive modality is used to stimulate healing, particularly in ligament, tendon, or bony structures. The Horse. 2015.

36. Lischer CJ, Ringer SK, Schnewlin M, et al. Treatment of chronic proximal suspensory desmitis in horses using focused electrohydraulic shockwave therapy. Schweiz Arch Tierheilkd 2006;148(10):561–8.

37. Hopper S. Treatment options for hind limb proximal suspensory desmitis.

38. Birch HL, Sinclair C, Goodchip A, et al. Tendon & ligament physiology. Equine Sports Medicine & Surgery 2014.

39. VersaTron. Available at: http://www.pulsevet.com/versatron-equine/about-versatron-equine.

40. Dakin SG, Dyson SJ, Murray RC, et al. Osseous abnormalities associated with collateral desmopathy of the distal interphalangeal joint. Part 2: treatment and outcome. Equine Vet J 2009;41(8):794–9.

41. Caminoto EH, Alves AL, Amorim RL, et al. Ultrastructural and immunocytochemical evaluation of the effects of extracorporeal shock wave treatment in the hind limbs of horses with experimentally induced suspensory ligament desmitis. Am J Vet Res 2005;66(5):892–6.

42. McClure SR, VanSickle D, Evans R, et al. The effects of extracorporeal shock-wave therapy on the ultrasonographic and histologic appearance of collagenase-induced equine forelimb suspensory ligament desmitis. Ultrasound Med Biol 2004;30(4):461–7.

43. Frisbie DD, Kawcak CE, McIlwraith CW. Evaluation of the effect of extracorporeal shock wave treatment on experimentally induced osteoarthritis in middle carpal joints of horses. Am J Vet Res 2009;70(4):449–54.

44. Godine RL. Low level laser therapy (LLLT) in veterinary medicine. Photomed Laser Surg 2014;32(1):1–2.
45. Dogan GE, Demir T, Orbak R. Effect of low-level laser on guided tissue regeneration performed with equine bone and membrane in the treatment of intrabony defects: a clinical study. Photomed Laser Surg 2014;32(4):226–31.
46. Marcos RL, Arnold G, Magnenet V, et al. Biomechanical and biochemical protective effect of low-level laser therapy for Achilles tendinitis. J Mech Behav Biomed Mater 2014;29:272–85.
47. Ron Riegel D. Laser therapy in equine practice. Vet Pract News 2012.
48. Laser O. Available at: http://www.omegalaser.co.uk/clinical_app_equinelaser therapy_landing.html.
49. Lasers A. 2015. Available at. http://www.apollopt.com/learn/blog/laser-therapy-for-the-equine-athlete.aspx.
50. Petersen SL, Botes C, Olivier A, et al. The effect of low level laser therapy (LLLT) on wound healing in horses. Equine Vet J 1999;31(3):228–31.
51. Moraes JM. Therapeutic ultrasound and low level laser in treatment of equine abscess. PUBVET 2014;8:16.
52. Alford CG. Equine distal limb wounds: new and emerging treatments. Compend Contin Educ Vet 2012;34(7):E5.
53. Cho HJ, Lim SC, Kim SG, et al. Effect of low-level laser therapy on osteoarthropathy in rabbit. In Vivo 2004;18(5):585–91.
54. Totosy de Zepetnek JO, Giangregorio LM, Craven BC. Whole body vibration as potential intervention for people with low bone mineral density and osteoporosis: a review. J Rehabil Res Dev 2009;46(4):529–42.
55. Knight M. Good vibrations. California Thoroghbred; 2009.
56. Vibratech. Available at: http://www.vibratech.co.il.
57. Carstanjen B, Balali M, Gajewski Z, et al. Short-term whole body vibration exercise in adult healthy horses. Pol J Vet Sci 2013;16(2):403–5.
58. Elmantaser M, McMillan M, Smith K, et al. A comparison of the effect of two types of vibration exercise on the endocrine and musculoskeletal system. J Musculoskelet Neuronal Interact 2012;12(3):144–54.
59. Kanter MM, Lesmes GR, Kaminsky LA, et al. Serum creatine kinase and lactate dehydrogenase changes following an eighty kilometer race. Relationship to lipid peroxidation. Eur J Appl Physiol Occup Physiol 1988;57(1):60–3.

Hyperbaric Oxygen Therapy in Equine Rehabilitation

Putting the Pressure on Disease

Dennis R. Geiser, DVM, CHT-V

KEYWORDS

- Hyperbaric • Oxygen • Rehabilitation • Equine

KEY POINTS

- There are several beneficial physiologic and therapeutic effects of hyperbaric oxygen therapy (HBOT).
- The indications list for the use of HBOT in the horse has been developed through extrapolation from a review of human indications and from anecdotal clinical experiences.
- Hyperbaric therapy is a safe treatment option with very few side effects when administered properly.

HISTORY OF HYPERBARIC MEDICINE

Oxygen was described around 1800, and in the mid 1960s, a project in pigs revealed that life could be maintained in an oxygen-pressurized chamber without the presence of red blood cells in the vasculature.[1] There was a surge of interest in treating animals with hyperbaric oxygen in the late 1990s with the production of large-animal hyperbaric chambers. That surge is now spilling over into the small animal world. There were many early animal hyperbaric treatments specifically for the generation of research data to benefit humans. However, there are little research data in the literature specifically directed at the clinical use of hyperbaric therapy in animals. Currently, the clinical use in horses is based on extrapolation from human and early animal research, from human clinical experiences, and from anecdotal clinical experiences and outcomes in horses. In general, the basic mechanisms of action and the physiologic effects of hyperbaric oxygen therapy (HBOT) are similar across domestic mammal species.

HOW IT WORKS

The ultimate goal of HBOT is to prevent, reduce, or eliminate tissue hypoxia by increasing the tissue oxygen concentration.[2–5] Varying degrees of tissue hypoxia

Regenerative Medicine Section, Department of Large Animal Clinical Sciences, College of Veterinary Medicine, University of Tennessee, 2407 River Drive, Knoxville, TN 37996-4545, USA
E-mail address: DGeiser@utk.edu

Vet Clin Equine 32 (2016) 149–157
http://dx.doi.org/10.1016/j.cveq.2015.12.010
0749-0739/16/$ – see front matter Published by Elsevier Inc.

vetequine.theclinics.com

occur in most disease situations. The creation of very high arterial and capillary oxygen concentrations drives oxygen into the tissues by developing a very large concentration gradient between the capillary and the tissue. This large gradient also increases the tissue oxygen diffusion distance. A 20-fold increase in arterial oxygen increases the diffusion distance approximately 4-fold.[6]

The blood oxygen concentration is normally composed of oxyhemoglobin plus the oxygen dissolved in the plasma (HbO_2 + Dissolved O_2 = Total Oxygen Content).[7] During HBOT, the potential is to increase the total blood oxygen content by as much as 15 times normal.[8] Even in the presence of decreased tissue blood flow, the use of HBOT can significantly increase tissue oxygenation.

The high plasma oxygen concentration is developed by 2 major pulmonary effects of HBOT: (1) increasing the density of oxygen molecules in the inspired gas, (2) further increasing the oxygen molecule density in the alveolus by decreasing alveolar volume. These 2 effects create a large concentration gradient between the alveolus and the pulmonary capillary blood, driving more oxygen into the plasma.

THE BENEFICIAL EFFECTS OF HYPERBARIC OXYGEN THERAPY

There are several beneficial physiologic and therapeutic effects of HBOT. These effects are summarized in **Table 1** .[8] HBOT is considered both a primary and an adjunctive therapy. In many cases, it is combined with other therapeutic modalities. Depending on the specific disease or injury, HBOT can be the factor that pushes the patient toward a positive outcome when standard therapeutic measures are ineffective. Hyperbaric therapy has cell/tissue salvage capabilities in any disease situation. Injured cells that are on the fence and could die or survive are pushed off the

Table 1
A summary of the general beneficial effects of hyperbaric oxygen therapy

Beneficial Effect	Reference
Increased tissue oxygen concentrations Support of aerobic metabolism Tissue salvage	4
Decreased blood flow in hyperoxic tissues but not hypoxic tissues Decreased edema Decreased cerebral blood flow & intracranial pressure Decreased cerebral edema	9–19
Supports effectiveness of some antibiotics Supports neutrophilic microbial killing Direct microbial killing or stasis	20–26
Increases antioxidant production Increases circulating stem cells Antagonizes lipid peroxidation Suppression of selected autoimmune responses	27–31
Decreases gas bubble size—embolism	32
Osteoclastic stimulation, bone remodeling, accelerated healing Accelerates bone repair	33–37
Decreases neutrophil–endothelial adherence	38–40
Stimulates fibroblasts and collagen production & remodeling Increases production and synergistic growth factor Support of neovascularization & epithelialization	41–47

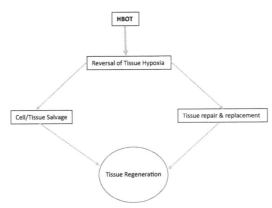

Fig. 1. The goal of HBOT is tissue regeneration, which includes the salvage of compromised tissue and the replacement of lost tissue through the reversal of tissue hypoxia.

fence to the survival side with the creation of a better, oxygenated environment. Hyperbaric therapy also plays a significant role in tissue regeneration following diseases and injuries, particularly if tissue hypoxia occurs during the disease process (**Fig. 1**). Although the scientific literature is all but devoid of quality evidence for HBOT use in

Table 2
Examples of some of the potential indications for hyperbaric oxygen therapy

Central Nervous System	Musculoskeletal System	Cardiovascular System
Cranial & spinal cord trauma	Tendonitis	Shock
Cerebral ischemia	Desmitis	Cardiac infarction
Compressive chord diseases	Periostitis	Acute anemia
Cortical blindness	Arthritis	Reperfusion disease
Peripheral nerve injury	Laminitis	Peripheral ischemia
Cerebral edema	Myositis	Carbon monoxide/dioxide
	Fracture	toxicity
		Lymphangitis

Respiratory System	Cutaneous System	Gastrointestinal System
Equine exercise induced	Compromised wounds	Ileus
pulmonary hemorrhage	Thermal burns	Pancreatitis
(EIPH)	Compromised grafts and flaps	Peritonitis
Pulmonary edema	Snake bite	Ulcers
Pleuritis	Spider bite	Reperfusion
Smoke inhalation		
Sinusitis		

Infectious	Genitourinary	
Osteomyelitis	Infertility	
Septic arthritis		
Septicemia		
Edotoxemia		
Rhodococcus equi		
Blastomycosis		
Lyme disease		
Anaerobic infections		
Intracranial and		
intra-abdominal abscess		
Equine protozoal myelitis		

Table 3
A summary of the potential beneficial effects and applications of hyperbaric oxygen therapy in equine rehabilitation

Indication	Supportive Mechanisms	Acute Effects	Clinical Impression
Tendon & ligament healing	Simulation of collagen production and deposition	Anti-inflammatory	Improved quality of healing
	Endogenous stem cell recruitment	Edema reduction	Reduction of time to return to function
	Growth factor stimulation and synergism	—	—
Cartilage and bone healing	Bone remodeling	Anti-inflammatory	Reduction of time to return to function
	Neovascularization	—	Transient analgesia
	Simulation of collagen production and deposition	—	—
	Stem cell recruitment	—	—
Wound healing	Stimulation of fibroblastic activity & collagen production	Resistance to infection: support of neutrophilic oxidative bacteria killing	Beneficial in compromised wounds
	Collagen synthesis and remodeling	Edema reduction	Beneficial for poor perfusion, edema, infection, large defects, failing graphs and flaps, envenomation, and burns
	Neovascularization	—	—
	Growth factor stimulation and synergism	—	—
	Proteoglycan synthesis	—	—
	Wound contraction	—	—
	Stem cell mobilization	—	—
	Epithelialization	—	—
Muscular conditions	Edema reduction: ↓compartment syndrome, re-establish microcirculation	Protects against reperfusion disease	Should be administered early in the disease process
	Reverse hypoxia, oxygen debt, & adverse biochemical alterations	—	—
	Support of intrinsic host factors	—	—
	Pain relief	—	—
Reperfusion disease	Decrease tissue hypoxia	—	Should be administered early in the disease process
	Decrease neutrophil to venule endothelial adhesion	—	—

(continued on next page)

Table 3
(continued)

Indication	Supportive Mechanisms	Acute Effects	Clinical Impression
Neurologic disease	Reduced cerebral blood flow	Reduced cerebral, chord, peripheral neuron edema	Effective in cases of cerebral edema and traumatic brain injuries
	Improved microcirculation	Prevention of tissue hypoxia & resultant adverse biochemical alterations (tissue and intracellular acidosis)	—
	Neuron rescue, prevention of disease progression	—	—
	Aids in nerve fiber regeneration	—	—
Intestinal adynamic ileus	Reduction of intestinal luminal diameter: physically and via gradients to remove intestinal gases	—	Begin administration within 12–18 h postoperative
	Decrease edema of the intestinal wall	—	—
	Reverse hypoxia, increase revascularization & repair	—	—
Postexercise recovery	Increase tissue and intracellular O_2	Anti-inflammatory	No evidence of early improved level of fitness for next competition
	Regeneration of high-energy compounds, ATP, AMP creatine phosphate	Pain management	—
	Normalization of acid base balance	—	—
	Aids in micromuscle fiber tear repair	—	—

the horse, there is a significant quantity of research in other species, from which one can extrapolate for the horse. Because of the amount of quality information available for other species, HBOT should be considered a very conventional therapy at this point.

Rehabilitation is a treatment or treatments designed to facilitate the process of recovery from injury, illness, or disease to as normal a condition as possible. Rehabilitation is commonly associated with musculoskeletal and/or neurologic injury or disease and is applied to normalize function as much as possible after the insult has occurred, and medical or surgical therapy has been completed. There are beneficial effects of HBOT that are directed at the specific disease or injury, and there are general effects that can be used to rehabilitate patients without specificity. These latter effects are those that support tissue salvage and regeneration and include endogenous stem cell release from the bone marrow, growth factor stimulation and synergism, decreased lipid peroxidation, vascular neogenesis, increased antioxidant production, increased collagen production and deposition, and reduction of tissue edema.

INDICATIONS FOR HYPERBARIC OXYGEN THERAPY

The indications list for the use of HBOT in the horse has been developed through extrapolation from a review of human indications and from anecdotal clinical experiences.[9] As with any therapy, HBOT is not a panacea. When properly applied, hyperbaric therapy can play a significant role in creating a successful outcome in many equine diseases, reducing recovery time, and improving the quality of healing and functionality. A partial list of indications in the horse is provided in **Table 2** .

HBOT in the rehabilitation of the equine patient can be used in synergism with the primary therapy or as an adjunct to improve healing and hasten recovery. For example, the use of HBOT plus antimicrobial therapy in a septic joint may improve the bacterial killing over the use of either treatment alone. On the other hand, the use of HBOT following surgical treatment of a subchondral bone cyst would be adjunctive to help stimulate remodeling and repair to achieve as near to normal articular surface as possible. A summary of potential beneficial effects of HBOT in equine rehabilitation is provided in **Table 3** .

APPLICATION OF HYPERBARIC OXYGEN THERAPY

Hyperbaric therapy is a safe treatment option with very few side effects when administered properly. Patients should be properly screened and examined for suitability. The use of HBOT should be based on a correlation of the pathophysiology of each

---

Box 1
Absolute and relative contraindications for hyperbaric oxygen therapy

Absolute contraindications

Untreated pneumothorax

Relative contraindications

Uncontrolled fever

Upper respiratory infections

Emphysema with CO_2 retention

Pulmonary bullae, cysts

Upper airway obstruction

Hypothermia

Uncontrolled hemorrhage

Uncontrolled seizure disorders

Absolute refers to those conditions for which the use of hyperbaric therapy could cause serious and potential fatal effects. Relative refers to those conditions, when present, that require a risk–benefit assessment and may delay or eliminate the use of hyperbaric therapy.
Data from Jain KK. Indications, contraindications and complications of HBO therapy. Textbook of hyperbaric medicine. 5th edition. Cambridge (United Kingdom): Hogrefe Publishing; 2009. p. 76; and Kindwall EP. Contraindications and side effects of hyperbaric oxygen treatment. In: Kindwall EP, Whelan HT, editors. Hyperbaric medicine practice. 3rd edition. Flagstaff (AZ): Best Publishing Company; 2008. p. 83–98.

specific disease or injury with the beneficial effects of HBOT. In addition, patients should be evaluated for their suitability to experience the pressurized environment. Assessments are performed based on history, diagnosis, current therapies, and a pretreatment physical examination. There are some contraindications for HBOT, which are listed in **Box 1**.

Protocols used to treat equine patients have been developed from clinical experience with extrapolation from the human hyperbaric medicine literature and past research in other species. In general, a single equine treatment would range in length from 45 to 60 minutes at the prescribed pressure. There would be an additional 10- to 15-minute pressurization time and a similar depressurization interval resulting in a total treatment time, surface to surface, of approximately 90 minutes. Treatment pressures range from 2.0 to 3.0 ATA. Maximum treatment pressure is 3 atmospheres absolute (ATA). Frequency and duration of the treatment plan will vary with the disease or injury being treated and the response to treatment. Routinely, patients are treated daily, but in some circumstances twice daily or an every-other-day treatment might be warranted. Total treatment days will vary from 3 to as many as 50 or more.

REFERENCES

1. Kindwall EP. A history of hyperbaric medicine. In: Kindwall EP, Whelan HT, editors. Hyperbaric medicine practice. 3rd edition. Flagstaff (AZ): Best Publishing Company; 2008. p. 1–19.
2. Kindwall EP. The physics of diving and hyperbaric pressures. In: Kindwall EP, Whelan HT, editors. Hyperbaric medicine practice. 3rd edition. Flagstaff (AZ): Best Publishing Company; 2008. p. 21–9.
3. Sheffield PJ, Smith APS. Physiological and pharmacological basis of hyperbaric oxygen therapy. In: Sheffield PJ, Smith APS, editors. Hyperbaric surgery: perioperative care. Flagstaff (AZ): Best Publishing Company; 2002. p. 63–74.
4. Jain KK. Physical, physiological, and biochemical aspects of hyperbaric oxygenation. In: Jain KK, editor. Textbook of hyperbaric medicine. 5th edition. Cambridge (United Kingdom): Hogrefe Publishing; 2009. p. 10–6.
5. Slovis N. Review of hyperbaric medicine. Journal of Equine Veterinary Science 2008;28:760–7.
6. Krogh A. The number and distribution of capillaries in muscle with calculations of the oxygen pressure.head necessary for supplying the tissue. J Physiol 1919;52: 409–15.
7. West JB. Respiratory physiology—the essentials. 9th edition. Baltimore (MD): Lippincott Williams and Wilkins; 2012. p. 77.
8. Hammarlund C. The physiologic effects of hyperbaric oxygen. In: Kindwall EP, Whelan HT, editors. Hyperbaric medicine practice. 1st edition. Flagstaff (AZ): Best Publishing Company; 1994. p. 37–65.
9. Bird AD, Tefler ABM. Effect of hyperbaric oxygen on limb circulation. Lancet 1965;1:355–6.
10. Lindblom L, Tuma RF, Arfors KE. Influence of oxygen on perfused capillary density and capillary red cell velocity in rabbit skeletal muscle. Microvasc Res 1980; 19:197–208.
11. Hordines C, Tyssebotn I. Effect of high ambient pressure and oxygen tension on organ blood flow in conscious rats. Undersea Biomed Res 1985;12:115–8.
12. Dooley JW, Mehm WJ. Noninvasive assessment of the vasoconstrictive effects of hyperoxygenation. Journal of Hyperbaric Medicine 1990;44(4):177–87.

13. Sirsjo A, Lewis D. Improved blood flow in post-ischemic skeletal muscle after hyperbaric oxygen treatment. Int J Microcirc Clin Exp 1990;1(Suppl):156.

14. Zamboni WA, Roth AC, Russell RC, et al. The effect of hyperbaric oxygen on reperfusion of ischemic axial skin flaps: a laser Doppler analysis. Ann Plast Surg 1992;28:339–41.

15. Ohta H, Yasuui N, Susuki N, et al. Measurement of cerebral blood flow under hyperbaric oxygenation in man – relationship between P_aO_2 and cerebral blood flow. In: Kindwal E, editor. Proceedings of the Eighth International Congress on Hyperbaric Medicine. Flagstaff (AZ): Best Publishing Co; 1987. p. 62–7.

16. Tomiyama Y, Jansen K, Brian JE, et al. Hemodilution, cerebral O_2 delivery and cerebral blood flow: a study using hyperbaric oxygen. Am J Physiol 1999;276(4): H1190–6.

17. Sukoff MH, Ragatz RE. Hyperbaric oxygenation for the treatment of acute cerebral edema. Neurosurgery 1982;10(1):29–38.

18. Ohta H. The effects of hyperoxemia on cerebral blood flow in normal humans. No To Shinkei 1986;38:949–59.

19. Nylander G, Lewis D, Nordstrom H, et al. Reduction of post-ischemic edema with hyperbaric oxygen. Plast Reconstr Surg 1985;76(4):596–603.

20. Park M. Effects of hyperbaric oxygen in infectious diseases: basic mechanisms. In: Kindwall EP, Whelan HT, editors. Hyperbaric medicine practice. 4th edition. Flagstaff (AZ): Best Publishing Company; 2004. p. 205–44.

21. Raffin TA, Simon LM, Braun D, et al. Effect of hyperoxia on the rate of generation of superoxide anions (SOA) in fee solution and in a cellular {alveolar macrophage (AM)} system. Clin Res 1977;45:157–66.

22. Park MK, Muhvich KH, Myers RAM, et al. Hyperoxia prolongs the aminoglycoside-induced postantibiotic effect in Pseudomonas aeruginosa. Antimicrob Agents Chemother 1991;35:691–5.

23. Reynolds AV, Hamilton-Miller JMT, Brumfitt W. Diminished effect of gentamycin under anaerobic or hypercapnic conditions. Lancet 1976;1(7957):447–9.

24. Gottlieb SF, Solosky JA, Aubrey R, et al. Synergistic action of increased oxygen tensions and PABA-folic acid antagonists on bacterial growth. Aerosp Med 1974; 45:829–33.

25. Babior BM. Oxygen-dependent microbial killing by phagocytes. N Engl J Med 1978;298:659–68.

26. Beaman L, Beaman BL. The role of oxygen and its derivatives in microbial pathogenesis and host defense. Annu Rev Microbiol 1984;38:27–48.

27. Dhar M, Neilsen N, Beatty K, et al. Equine peripheral blood-derived mesenchymal stem cells: isolation, identification, trilineage differentiation and the effect of hyperbaric oxygen treatment. Equine Vet J 2012;44:600–5.

28. Thom SR. CO poisoning in a rat model: physiological correlation with clinical events and the effects of HBO [abstract only]. Undersea Biomed Res 1989; 16(Suppl):51–2.

29. Warren J, Sacksteder MR, Thuning CA. Oxygeb immunosuppression: modification of experimental allergic encephalomyelitis in rodents. J Immunol 1978;121: 315–20.

30. Felfmeyer JJ, Boswell RN, Brown M, et al. The effects of hyperbaric oxygen on the immunologic status of healthy human subjects. In: Kindwall EP, editor. Proceedings of the Eighth International Congress on Hyperbaric Medicine. Flagstaff (AZ): Best Publishing Co; 1987. p. 41–6.

31. Thom SR, Elbukin ME. Oxygen dependent antagonism of lipid peroxidation. Free Radic Biol Med 1991;10:413.

32. Hammarlund C. The physiologic effects of hyperbaric oxygenation. In: Kindwall EP, Whelan HT, editors. Hyperbaric medicine practice. 4th edition. Flagstaff (AZ): Best Publishing Company; 2004. p. 38–9.
33. Yablon IG, Cruess RL. The effect of hyperbaric oxygen on fracture healing in rats. J Surg Res 1968;8(8):373–8.
34. Esterhai JL, Clark J, Morton HE, et al. The effect of hyperbaric oxygen on oxygen tension within the medullary canal in the rabbit tibia model. J Orthop Res 1986;4: 330–6.
35. Barth E, Sullivan T, Berg E. Animal model for evaluating bone repair with and without adjunctive hyperbaric oxygen therapy (HBO): comparing dose schedules. J Invest Surg 1990;3:387–92.
36. Hunt TK, Niinikoski J, Zederfeldt BH, et al. Oxygen in wound healing enhancement; cellular effects of oxygen. In: Davis JC, Hunt TK, editors. Hyperbaric oxygen therapy. Bethesda (MD): Undersea Medical Society, Inc; 1977. p. 111–2.
37. Hunt TK, Pai MP. The effect of varying ambient oxygen tensions on wound metabolism and collagen synthesis. Surg Gynecol Obstet 1972;135:756–8.
38. Zamboni WA, Roth AC, Bergman BA, et al. Morphological analysis of the microcirculation during reperfusion of ischemic skeletal muscle and the effect of hyperbaric oxygen. Plast Reconstr Surg 1993;91:1110–23.
39. Larson JL, Stephenson LL, Zamboni WA. The effects of HBO on PMN expression of CD18 in a rat model of ischemia reperfusion (IR). Undersea Hyperb Med 1998; 25.
40. Banick PD, Chen Q, Xu YA, et al. Nitric oxide inhibits neutrophil beta 2 integrin function by inhibiting membrane-associated cyclic GMP synthesis. J Cell Physiol 1997;172:12–24.
41. Tompach PC, Lew D, Stoll JL. Cell response to hyperbaric oxygen treatment. Int J Oral Maxillofac Surg 1997;26:82–6.
42. Zhao LL, Davidson JD, Wee SC, et al. Effect of hyperbaric oxygen and growth factors on rabbit ischemic ulcers. Arch Surg 1994;129:1043–9.
43. Frank S, Stallmeyer B, Kampfer H, et al. Nitric oxide triggers enhanced induction of vascular endothelial growth factor expression in cultured keratinocytes (HaCaT) and during cutaneous wound repair. Arterioscler Thromb Vasc Biol 2000; 20(6):1512–20.
44. Bonomo SR, Davidson JD, Yu Y, et al. Hyperbaric oxygen as a signal transducer: upregulation of platelet derived growth factor beta receptor in the presence of HBO and PDGF. Arch Surg 1994;129(10):1043–9.
45. Bayati S, Russell RC, Roth AC. Stimulation of angiogenesis to improve viability of prefabricated flaps. J Clin Immunol 1997;17(2):154–9.
46. Gimball M, Hunt TK. Wound healing and hyperbaric oxygenation. In: Kindwall EP, Whelan HT, editors. Hyperbaric medicine practice. 3rd edition. Flagstaff (AZ): Best Publishing Company; 2008. p. 169–94.
47. Jain KK. HBO therapy in wound healing, plastic surgery, and dermatology. In: Jain KK, editor. Textbook of hyperbaric medicine. 5th edition. Cambridge (United Kingdom): Hogrefe Publishing; 2009. p. 157–76.

Controlled Exercise in Equine Rehabilitation

 CrossMark

Elizabeth J. Davidson, DVM

KEYWORDS

- Controlled exercise • Equine • Rehabilitation

KEY POINTS

- Controlled exercise is a fundamental and critical component of any rehabilitation program for the equine athlete.
- An ideal controlled exercise program complements and enhances the normal tissue reparative response after the injury.
- The best program is designed after accurate diagnosis regarding injury type and severity is determined and periodically adapted based on the quality of tissue healing.
- In general, a program starts with complete rest followed by stall rest with gradual and systematic increases in exercise intensity.
- A well designed, injury-directed, controlled exercise program enhances tissue healing during rehabilitation.

INTRODUCTION

Controlled exercise therapy is a standard fundamental part of almost all rehabilitation programs. It is time honored, deeply engrained in tradition, and considered routine practice for the injured equine athlete. Despite being the backbone of a rehabilitation program, there are few controlled studies in horses investigating the therapeutic effects of controlled exercise on musculoskeletal injuries. Most of what is known and practiced is based on intuition, common sense, and experience.[1]

In the human literature, therapeutic exercise is an effective and beneficial treatment for a variety of musculoskeletal problems.[2,3] Controlled mobilization (exercise) after injury produces better quality healing of muscles, tendons, and ligaments.[4] The goals of a rehabilitation program are to prevent further injury and enhance tissue healing. An ideal program relies on the basic understanding of the normal tissue response after the injury.

TISSUE HEALING AFTER INJURY

Tissue healing is an intricate process, and the rate and quality of healing are related to the intrinsic properties of the injured tissue. The process is complex and highly

Department of Clinical Studies, University of Pennsylvania, New Bolton Center, 382 West Street Road, Kennett Square, PA 19348, USA
E-mail address: ejdavid@vet.upenn.edu

Vet Clin Equine 32 (2016) 159–165
http://dx.doi.org/10.1016/j.cveq.2015.12.012
0749-0739/16/$ – see front matter © 2016 Elsevier Inc. All rights reserved.

susceptible to failure, especially when postinjury regimens are too much too soon for the healing tissue. Equally important is not prolonging the healing process. Huge economic costs are attributed to loss of use of the horse[5] and protracted recuperation periods add to these financial losses. Having an understanding of the phases of wound healing enhances the clinician's ability to apply an appropriate controlled exercise program in alignment with the healing process of the injured tissue.

In general, tissue healing is divided into predicable phases: hemostasis, inflammation, proliferation, and maturation. This basic principle applies to all tissues. Within the first minutes of injury, platelet and accompanying platelet activation result in clot formation. The formed fibrin acts as a glue to prevent further bleeding. Once hemostasis is achieved, blood vessels dilate, and there is an influx of erythrocytes and inflammatory cells, particularly neutrophils cells. In the next 24 to 48 hours, monocytes and macrophages predominate, and phagocytosis of necrotic material occurs. Vasoactive and chemotactic factors are released with increased vascular permeability, initiation of angiogenesis, stimulation of cell proliferation, and recruitment of more inflammatory cells. This acute inflammatory phase occurs during the first 7 days after injury.

The proliferative phase (about days 7–21) is characterized by proliferation of fibroblasts, myofibroplasts, synovial cells, and capillaries. Capillary beds start to grow; fibroblasts produce new collagen, and granulation tissue replaces the originally formed clot. Myofibroblastic activity causes wound contraction, and depending on the size of the injury, wound closure usually occurs within 5 to 8 days in muscle and 3 to 6 weeks in tendon and ligaments. During this stage of healing, the immature connective tissue is thin and unorganized. It is extremely fragile and easily injured if overstressed. Proper growth and arrangement of the healing tissue can be stimulated by tensile loading in alignment of normal stresses of the injured injury. At the same time, adhesion formation to surrounding tissues can be minimized.

Maturation and remodeling start at around day 21 after injury and continues for the next weeks to months. Collagen fibers start to reorganize themselves into normal orientation and begin to withstand normal stresses. The duration of the maturation process depends on the type of tissue injured. The entire process takes months and up to 1 to 2 years for tendon and ligament injuries.

Specific Tissue Injuries

Muscle

Muscle injury occurs through a variety of mechanisms, including direct trauma (lacerations, contusions, and strains) and indirect causes (ischemia and neurologic dysfunction). The different phases of healing occurring within the damaged muscle are similar among various types of muscle injuries, but the functional recovery of the injured muscle varies from one type of injury to another. Mechanical trauma destroys the integrity of the myofiber plasma membrane, resulting in local swelling and hematoma formation. Blood vessel invasion, mononuclear cells, activated macrophages, and T-lymphocytes closely follow. Muscle regeneration starts 7 to 10 days after injury, peaks at 2 weeks, and then decreases 3 to 4 weeks after injury. The formation of scar tissue (fibrosis) begins between 2 to 3 weeks after injury. Scar tissue contraction and reorganization, and the recovery of muscle function, occur over time. Immobilization is indicated for the first 4 to 7 days after injury[6] and helps to avoid rerupture of muscle fibers during acute phases of healing. This stage is followed by the gradual introduction of a controlled exercise program. A progressively intensified exercise program optimizes the healing by restoring the strength of the injured muscle and preventing muscle atrophy. Minor muscle injuries will heal within 4 weeks, whereas severe muscle injuries can take months before complete return of function is obtained.

Bone

Unlike other tissues, bone has the amazing ability to heal itself with similar tissue. The resultant healed bone can be as strong as or stronger than its original form. Its healing process involves inflammation, soft callus, hard callus, followed by bone remodeling. Soft fibrous or fibrocartilaginous callus formation is rapid and provides a scaffold for circulation and endosteal bone formation. The amount of activity influences the amount of callus formation. High motion results in large callus, and excessive movement (ie, uncontrolled exercise in turn-out paddock) can result in complete callus disruption and loss of bone union. As healing progresses, hard callus begins to form, which corresponds to clinical and radiographic fracture healing. In the mature adult horse, the entire process takes about 4 months. Over the next months to years, bone continues to remodel, adapting to the loads placed on it (Wolff law).

Tendon and ligament

Tendons and ligaments heal similarly. Shortly after insult, tenocytes migrate to the injury site from adjacent tendon/ligament cells and via the local blood supply. Collagen synthesis is initiated and collagen fibers are oriented perpendicular to the long axis of the tendon. After approximately 6 weeks, modeling and remodeling occur, and collagen orientation becomes parallel to the longitudinal axis of the tendon. Ultimate maturation of tendon/ligament fibers depends on sufficient and appropriate physiologic loading. Prolonged tendon immobilization reduces water and proteoglycan content. Unstressed collagen remains haphazard in organization and weaker than organized fiber alignment,[7] resulting in lower tensile strength and failure at lower strains. Mechanical stress is required to promote appropriate orientation and remodeling of collagen into mature, strong, and optimized tissue. Controlled exercise during the chronic remodeling phase helps to promote this conversion and improves the mechanical properties of the healed tendon. The quality of the longitudinal fiber pattern has been linked to prognosis for return to work.[8] Conversely, excessive loading may delay or disrupt the healing process. If the cross-sectional area of the healing tendon increases by more than 10%, the exercise level should be reduced.[9] For horses with tendon/ligament injuries, the duration of the controlled exercise program is critical, and horses rested for less than 6 months have a poorer prognosis.[10] Unfortunately, injured tendons and ligaments never regain normal functionality, and reinjury is common even in the appropriately rehabilitated tendon or ligament.

Cartilage

It is well known that cartilage has a limited ability to heal.[11] Clot formation does not occur nor does recruitment of neutrophils or macrophages. Healthy adjacent chondrocytes have a limited capacity to induce healing, and cartilaginous defects rarely resolve. Deeper cartilage lesions involving the subchondral bone allows for the formation of fibrin-fibronectin clot, which results in inflammation and granulation phases of healing to occur. The biochemical composition of repair tissue is more akin to fibrous than hyaline cartilage, and its resultant mechanical properties are significantly inferior to the latter. The therapeutic effects of exercise on induced cartilage lesions include thicker repair tissue, increased glycosaminoglycan content, and less bone remodeling with exercise.[12,13] However, repetitive or sudden mechanical impact during exercise is a significant risk factor for joint abnormality, and the equine carpal osteochondral fragment combined with exercise is a predictable and well-accepted model for osteoarthritis.[14]

PRESCRIPTION FOR CONTROLLED EXERCISE PROGRAM

Before designing an appropriate controlled exercise program, a complete and accurate diagnosis is essential because an incorrect diagnosis leads to an inappropriate and potentially detrimental after-injury therapy program. Without a proper diagnosis and treatment, there is a higher risk for reinjury or inability to return to athletic function. Diagnosis includes determining what tissue is injured and the severity of the injury. Many horses suffer from complex and/or multiple limb injuries, and every effort should be made to fully understand the extent of the horse's injury before instituting a therapy program. For instance, rehabilitation following a sesamoid fracture will have a poor result if concomitant suspensory desmitis is not recognized and also treated. In this horse, early return to uncontrolled exercise following fracture repair may result in incomplete healing or reinjury of the suspensory ligament, leading to prolonged and potentially permanent loss of athletic use of the horse.

Other considerations when planning a controlled exercise program include the horse's tolerability of extensive periods of stall rest. Despite owner's antics, horses will adapt and endure months of stall rest without negative psychological effects.[15] Good management practices such as adequate ventilation and clean bedding are indicated especially for prolonged periods of confinement. Adequate hoof care is also important and should not be neglected during the recuperation period. Cardiac and muscle function do not undergo significant deconditioning for at least 4 weeks after injury, and therefore, horses with minor injuries may return to full function with no or minimal loss of fitness. Last, stall confinement combined with controlled exercise in the form of hand walking or walking under saddle is preferred over turn-out, whereby uncontrolled horses frequently run, buck, spin, and slide. Excessive forces on healing tissues are detrimental to the repair process, resulting in inadequate or improper scar tissue formation.

The ideal after-injury rehabilitation program is formulated to complement and enhance the healing process. The basic principle is to reduce the force and strain on injured tissue while the normal reparative process proceeds. Immediately after injury, protection of the affected tissue is necessary. Complete rest (stall confinement) and, when indicated, cold therapy (ice) and compression (bandage) are recommended to minimize pain and promote healing. For the next 1 to 3 weeks, injury protection is maintained to prevent reinjury. Stall rest combined with short periods of walking is indicated. As tissue healing continues, a controlled exercise program is instituted that enhances the repair process. Extended periods of immobilization can have deleterious effects on musculoskeletal systems and should be avoided.[16] Controlled movement of muscles, tendons, ligaments, and joints improves the

Table 1
Controlled exercise protocol following muscle injury

Duration After Injury	Controlled Exercise (Daily)
Week 1	Stall rest
Week 2	Stall rest, walk 15 min
Week 3	Stall rest, walk 30 min
Week 4	Stall rest, walk 30 min, trot 5 min
Week 5	Stall rest, walk 20 min, trot 10 min
Week 6	Stall rest, walk 20 min, trot 20 min
Week 7	Stall rest, walk 20 min, trot 20 min, canter 5 min
Week 8+	Small paddock turn out (20 × 20 ft), gradually increase exercise level gradually to full training

Table 2
Controlled exercise protocol following bone injury

Duration After Injury	Controlled Exercise (Daily)
Weeks 1–4	Stall rest
Weeks 5–6	Stall rest, walk 15 min
Weeks 7–8[a]	Stall rest, walk 30 min
Weeks 9–16	Small paddock turn out (20 × 20 ft)
Weeks 16+	Gradually increase exercise level to full training

[a] Radiographic evaluation to assess bone healing after 8 weeks and before small paddock turn out.

orientation of collagen fibers to withstand the tensile forces and prevents tissue atrophy.

The controlled exercise program is designed based on the type and severity of the injury. General recommendations are included (**Tables 1–3**); however, an ideal program is based on the individual horse's physical impairment. As the injury continues to heal, gradual incremental increases in activity are instituted. For best results, regular and periodic veterinary examination combined with diagnostic imaging, when

Table 3
Controlled exercise protocol following tendon or ligament injury

Duration After Injury	Controlled Exercise (Daily)
Weeks 1–2	Stall rest
Weeks 3–4	Stall rest, walk 5 min
Weeks 5–6	Stall rest, walk 10 min
Weeks 7–8	Stall rest, walk 15 min
Weeks 9–10[a]	Stall rest, walk 20 min
Weeks 11–12	Stall rest, walk 25 min
Weeks 13–14	Stall rest, walk 30 min
Weeks 15–16	Stall rest, walk 35 min
Weeks 17–18[a]	Stall rest, walk 40 min
Weeks 19–20	Stall rest, walk 40 min, trot 2 min
Weeks 21–22	Stall rest, walk 35 min, trot 5 min
Weeks 23–24	Stall rest, walk 30 min, trot 10 min
Weeks 25–26[a]	Stall rest, walk 25 min, trot 15 min
Weeks 27–28	Stall rest, walk 20 min, trot 20 min
Weeks 29–30	Stall rest, walk 20 min, trot 20 min, canter 1 min
Weeks 31–32	Stall rest, walk 20 min, trot 20 min, canter 5 min
Weeks 33–34[a]	Stall rest, walk 20 min, trot 20 min, canter 10 min
Weeks 35–36	Stall rest, walk 15 min, trot 20 min, canter 15 min
Weeks 37–38	Stall rest, walk 10 min, trot 20 min, canter 20 min
Weeks 39–42[a]	Small paddock turn out (20 × 20 ft), full flat work, no speed work or jumping
Weeks 42+	Small paddock turn out (20 × 20 ft), full flat work, gradually introduce speed work or jumping

[a] Lameness and ultrasound examination. The horse continues with program with improved assessment.

appropriate, is recommended every 2 to 3 months. The frequency, amount, and type of exercise are prescribed and adjusted throughout the entire healing process. Horses with improved lameness and imaging scores during follow-up examinations continue with gradual increases in exercise intensity. Decreasing or temporarily discontinuing exercise is indicated for horses with lameness and/or lack of healing based on imaging. Specific recommendations, such as how many minutes of walk and trot, are greatly appreciated by the client.

The controlled exercise program may require modifications depending on the horse handler's ability, the facilities, and the horse's disposition. Although ridden exercise or caged horse walkers (equine exercisers) are preferred over paddock rest, the use of a small paddock (12 × 12 ft) to inhibit running and other uncontrolled activities may be a suitable compromise. Ancillary aids including shoeing modifications, anti-inflammatory medications, pain relief, and leg bandaging are also beneficial. Exercises that result in swelling and/or lameness are contradicted and the program should be modified accordingly.

REFERENCES

1. Grant BE. Rest and rehabilitation. In: Ross MW, Dyson SJ, editors. Diagnosis and management of lameness in the horse. 2nd edition. St. Louis: Elsevier; 2011. p. 877–80.
2. Smidt N, Henrica CWV, Bouter LM, et al. Effectiveness of exercise therapy: a best-evidence summary of systematic reviews. Aust J Physiother 2005;51:71–85.
3. Taylor NF, Dodd KJ, Sheild N, et al. Therapeutic exercise in physiotherapy practice is beneficial: a summary of systemic reviews 2002-2005. Aust J Physiother 2007;53:7–16.
4. Kannus P, Parkkari J, Narvinen TLN, et al. Basic science and clinical studies coincide: active treatment approach is needed after sports injury. Scand J Med Sci Sports 2003;13:150–4.
5. Anon (2001) National economic cost of equine lameness, colic, and equine protozoal myeloencephalitis in the United States. In USDA: APHIS:VS, National Health Monitoring System. Information Sheet. Fort Collins. #N348.1001.
6. Jarvinen TAH, Jarvinen M, Kalimo H. Regeneration of skeletal muscle after the injury. Muscles Ligaments Tendons J 2013;3(4):337–45.
7. Sharma P, Maffulli N. Tendon injury and tendinopathy: healing and repair. J Bone Joint Surg Am 2005;87(1):187–202.
8. Reef VB, Genovese RL, Davis WM. Initial long-term results of horses with superficial digital flexor tendonitis treated with intralesional beta-aminoproprionitrile fumarate. Proc Am Assoc Equine Pract 1997;43:301–5.
9. Smith RKW. Pathophysiology of tendon injury. In: Ross MW, Dyson SJ, editors. Diagnosis and management of lameness in the horse. 2nd edition. St Louis (MO): Elsevier; 2011. p. 706–26.
10. Dowling BA, Dart AJ, Hodgson DR, et al. Superficial digital flexor tendonitis in the horse. Equine Vet J 2000;32:369–78.
11. Hunzike EB. Articular cartilage repair: basic science and clinical progress. A review of the current status and prospects. Osteoarthritis Cartilage 2001;10:432–63.
12. French DA, Barber SM, Leach D, et al. The effect of exercise on the healing of articular cartilage defects in the equine carpus. Vet Surg 1989;18:312–21.

13. Foland JW, McIlwraith CW, Trotter GW, et al. Effect of betamethasone and exercise on equine carpal joints with osteochondral fragments. Vet Surg 1994;23: 369–76.
14. McIlwraith CW. The horse as a model of naturally occurring osteoarthritis. Bone Joint Res 2012;11:297–309.
15. Houpt K, Houpt TR, Johnson JL, et al. The effect of exercise deprivation on the behavior and physiology of straight stall confined pregnant mares. Anim Welf 2001;10:257–67.
16. Paulekas R, Haussler KK. Principles and practice of therapeutic exercise for horses. J Equine Vet Sci 2009;29(12):870–93.

Practical Rehabilitation and Physical Therapy for the General Equine Practitioner

CrossMark

Andris J. Kaneps, DVM, PhD

KEYWORDS

- Equine • Rehabilitation • Sports medicine • Physical therapy

KEY POINTS

- Physical treatment and rehabilitation play major roles in recovery and maintenance of the equine athlete, and many therapeutic measures are accessible by the veterinarian in general practice.
- The basis for any treatment regimen is an accurate diagnosis with measurable outcome parameters.
- The general practitioner may readily use treatments from the electrophysical modality group and make recommendations for appropriate rehabilitation exercise.
- Consulting with specialist veterinarians trained in equine rehabilitation therapy or physical therapists trained in equine therapy is necessary for making appropriate treatment decisions.

Physical treatment and rehabilitation of horses is a major contributor to a successful outcome of surgical or medical therapy. It may also be the primary therapy when a horse is competing under *Federation Equestre Internationale* or other competition regulations that prohibit the use of medications.

Application of these techniques requires knowledge of indications, methods of treatment, and end points. For the general equine practitioner, rehabilitation therapy should be collaboration with a veterinarian or physical therapist trained in equine techniques. A veterinary technician trained and certified in an equine rehabilitation therapy program is also a useful resource.

The basis for any treatment regimen is an accurate diagnosis. Using lameness as an example, the practitioner must clearly identify the specific anatomic location, tissue injury, and other ancillary factors that are contributing to the gait abnormality. High-quality imaging is necessary to make the diagnosis and is used to monitor the response to treatment. For example, characteristics of the injured tissue, such as

Disclosure statement: The author has nothing to disclose.
Kaneps Equine Sports Medicine and Surgery, LLC, 68 Grover Street, Beverly, MA 01915, USA
E-mail address: AJKANEPS@KANEPSEQUINE.COM

Vet Clin Equine 32 (2016) 167–180
http://dx.doi.org/10.1016/j.cveq.2015.12.001
0749-0739/16/$ – see front matter © 2016 Elsevier Inc. All rights reserved.

cross-sectional area, fiber pattern, and echogenicity, should be recorded for ultrasonographic evaluations. Other measurements may be made at the injury site and recorded for future use during rehabilitation. Examples include circumference of a swollen injury site, range of motion/degrees of flexion measured with a goniometer, and response to deep palpation over an injury site (subjective assessment or objective measurement using algometry). A complete diagnosis may require referral to an equine imaging center that has computed tomography, magnetic resonance, or scintigraphy imaging capabilities.

This article reviews common therapeutic modalities accessible to the equine practitioner.

THERMAL THERAPY

One of the most accessible and time-tested methods of physical treatment is thermal therapy (**Table 1**). Heat or cold may be administered to horses using many modalities and can range from simply applying water from a hose to cooling tissues with compression using therapeutic boots.

Cold Therapy

The major physiologic benefits of cold therapy are reduced local circulation, tissue swelling, and pain sensation.[1,2] These benefits are most effective early in the period following injury or surgery. The primary effect of local cold application is to constrict blood vessels and reduce tissue temperature. Reduced blood flow will reduce edema, hemorrhage, and extravasation of inflammatory cells. Cold reduces tissue metabolism and may inhibit the effect of inflammatory mediators and slow enzyme systems. Cyclical rebound vasodilatation is another response to cold therapy. After a minimum of 15 minutes of cold therapy that results in tissue temperatures from 10°C to 15°C, cycles of vasoconstriction and vasodilatation occur. Vasodilatation associated with cold therapy may help further resolve tissue edema. Analgesia is a significant effect of cold therapy.

Cold therapy is indicated in acute musculoskeletal injuries and following surgical procedures to reduce edema, slow the inflammatory response, and reduce pain. It is particularly effective during the first 24 to 48 hours after injury or surgery. Cold immersion of the distal limbs is also effective in reducing severity of laminitis by

Table 1			
Thermal therapy indications, methods, and physiologic responses			
Therapy Type	**Indications**	**Methods of Application**	**Responses to Treatment**
Cold	• Acute injury (first 24–48 h) • Pain reduction	• Ice water immersion • Ice surface application • Cold packs	• Restricts blood flow • Reduces metabolism • Reduces activity of inflammatory enzymes • Reduces pain
Heat	• Chronic injury (after 72 h) • Enhance tissue stretching • Enhance healing response	• Warm water from hose • Hot packs • Leg sweat • Therapeutic ultrasound	• Increases blood flow • Increases metabolism • Increases activity of tissue enzymes • Relaxes muscle spasm • Reduces pain • Increased tissue extensibility

decreasing the activity of laminar matrix metalloproteinases and causing laminar vasoconstriction when applied during the developmental phase.[3]

Cold may be applied by ice water immersion, application of ice packs or cold packs, cold water from a hose, and ice water–charged circulating bandages or boots. The most beneficial therapeutic effects of cold occur at tissue temperatures between 15°C and 19°C (59°F to 66°F).[1] Average time of cold application is 20 to 30 minutes. Treatments are best repeated every 2 to 4 hours during the first 48 to 72 hours of injury or surgery if the goal is to reduce tissue inflammation. Direct contact of ice water with the skin is the most effective method of cold therapy. Buckets or turbulator boots may be used depending on the treatment site. If immersion therapy is used immediately following surgery, the wound must be protected with a water impervious barrier.

To prevent or treat laminitis, continuous cold therapy is applied to the distal limbs using plastic bags filled with ice, ice water immersion, or commercial cold therapy boots. A simple method to effectively cool the distal limb using a bag-within-a bag that contains an ice water slurry has been reported.[4] Empty 5-L fluid bags are placed on the distal limb and secured with ice between the bags (**Fig. 1**). This technique effectively reduces tissue temperatures for a prolonged period of time. Ice water immersion of the equine digit for 30 minutes resulted in significant decreases in laminar temperatures.[4] Comparison of laminar and venous temperatures was made between ice water immersion in vinyl boots, ice water slurry in plastic bags, and application of malleable cold packs. Ice water immersion and the ice water slurry in bags were comparable in reducing measured temperatures, whereas cold packs did not substantially reduce temperatures.[4] The successful cooling of blood and laminae in a hoof at risk for laminitis reduces the likelihood of clinical laminitis signs of inflammation, pain, and distal phalanx displacement.[3] Cooling of a hoof that has clinical signs of laminitis will reduce the degree of inflammation and pain present.

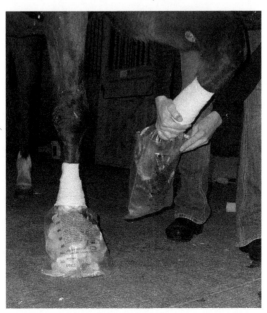

Fig. 1. Application of 2 fluid administration bags, with ice water slurry between them, is an effective method to cool the distal limb.

Boots that connect to a cold source and circulate fluid through them are also very effective at chilling tissue (**Fig. 2**). Systems are available with a variety of boot configurations for different portions of the limb, making effective cold therapy logistically very simple (Game Ready, Concord, CA, USA). Some of the systems also provide compression and may be used for cold or heat therapy.

Cold therapy may also be applied by running a cold water hose on the target site. This method is very practical, but is not as effective at reducing tissue temperatures as ice water immersion.[5] The physical pressure from a hose with a spray nozzle is helpful in resolving edema and in debriding wounds.

Heat Therapy

The major physiologic benefits of heat therapy are increased local circulation, muscle relaxation (and therefore, reduction of muscle spasms and associated pain), and increased tissue extensibility.[1,2] Increased local blood flow mobilizes tissue metabolites, increases tissue oxygenation, and increases the metabolic rate of cells and enzyme systems. Metabolic rate increases 2 to 3 times for a tissue temperature increase of 10°C.[1] These responses to heat therapy are especially beneficial for wound

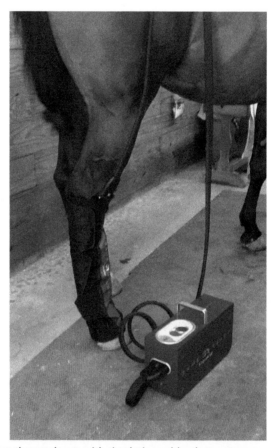

Fig. 2. Compression therapy boots with circulating cold or hot water are useful for treatment of cellulitis, lymphangitis, and other inflammatory conditions of the limb (Game Ready, Concord, CA).

healing. Increased blood flow and vascular permeability may promote resorption of edema, which is a common reason for heat application in horses. Heat application also decreases pain. Soft tissues may be stretched more effectively when they are warm. Heat decreases tissue viscosity and increases tissue elasticity. Low-load, prolonged stretching of tissues heated from 40°C to 45°C (104°F to 113°F) results in increased extensibility of tendons, joint capsules, and muscles.[1,2]

Heat is best applied after acute inflammation has subsided. It is useful for reducing muscle spasms and pain because of musculoskeletal injuries. Heat therapy can be used to increase joint and tendon mobility, particularly when heat is applied before active stretching. Heat may benefit recovery of localized soft tissue injuries by accelerating the healing response.

Superficial heat is most commonly applied using hot packs and hydrotherapy. These modalities provide heat penetration to approximately 1 cm deep to the skin. The most profound physiologic effects of heat occur when tissue temperatures are raised to 40°C to 45°C (104°F to 113°F).[1,2] Tissue temperatures greater than 45°C may result in pain and tissue damage. For deeper tissues, such as tendon or muscle, 15 to 30 minutes is required to elevate tissue temperature to the therapeutic range. When using heat sources warmer than 45°C, the source must be wrapped in several layers of moist towels before application. Heat from these sources is usually applied for 20 to 30 minutes. Warm water is probably the most accessible method of heat therapy. Methods of application include the use of a hose, wet towels, water immersion in a bucket, turbulator boot, and circulating treatment system. A rule of thumb is that water as hot as your hand can comfortably stand has a temperature of 38°C to 41°C (101°F to 105°F). However, tissue heated by water at this temperature may only reach the lowest tissue therapeutic range. Therefore, the target temperature should be above this level, but as mentioned earlier, horses will commonly experience discomfort with water 45°C and warmer.

Heat may be used to relax tight muscles in the back before exercise. Simply using a thick fleece blanket or exercise rug can be used to relax muscle spasm and prepare the back for stretching exercises or riding (**Fig. 3**).

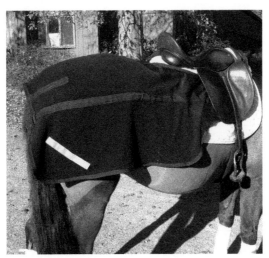

Fig. 3. A fleece exercise blanket may be used to warm the back before and during exercise to relieve muscle spasm.

The use of magnetic blankets has been another treatment method used to treat muscle stiffness and soreness by increasing local blood flow. However, a study of a static magnetic field blanket on back muscle blood flow, skin temperature, mechanical nociceptive threshold, or behavior in normal horses failed to find any changes following a 60-minute treatment.[6]

THERAPEUTIC ULTRASOUND

Therapeutic ultrasound may be used to stimulate healing, for pain relief, for reduction of tissue edema, and for reduction of fibrous scar.[7,8] The sound waves of therapeutic ultrasound result in micromassage of tissues and acoustic streaming of fluids and ions.[7] These effects result in compression and expansion of tissues and tissue fluids that may improve tissue healing. Heating of muscle has been identified in the dog and human, but not in the horse.[2,9–11] Horse tendons are effectively heated with ultrasound.[11]

Treatment is commonly performed once or twice daily for 10 to 14 days. The hair must be clipped, and coupling gel must be used to provide good contact between the transducer and the skin. In horses, standard therapeutic ultrasound treatment is usually conducted with a 1-MHz transducer for deepest penetration (2.5–5 cm depth) and 3-mHz (1–2.5 cm depth) for superficial penetration. Energy levels administered are 1 to 2 W/cm^2, with a continuous wave for 10 minutes.[12,13] The transducer should be slowly moved throughout the treatment area. Pulsed wave may be used over a bony prominence to reduce discomfort. The ability to manipulate the transducer and adjustment of treatment output for specific circumstances makes traditional therapeutic ultrasound the most versatile means for applying this modality (**Fig. 4**).

Low-intensity ultrasound may be applied for 2 to 3 hours of treatment for acute injuries and 4 to 6 hours once daily for chronic injuries. The device does not have adjustable settings with output set at 2.75 MHz at 0.85 W/cm^2. For accessible anatomic locations, the device is placed on the limb for the appropriate treatment time (UltrOZ; ZetrOZ LLC, Trumbull, CT, USA) (**Fig. 5**).

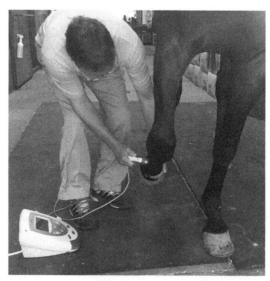

Fig. 4. Traditional therapeutic ultrasound allows for manipulation of the transducer over a variety of anatomic sites and for adjustment of treatment output, yet requires a trained individual to administer treatment.

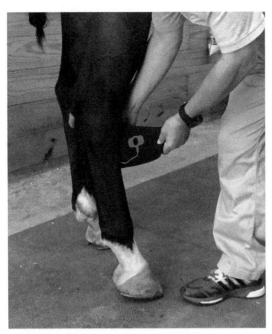

Fig. 5. Low-level therapeutic ultrasound with preset wavelength and power output is used to administer therapy over several hours. The transducer (*black disc within blue holder*) is attached to an elastic sleeve that is secured over the treatment site.

EXTRACORPOREAL SHOCK WAVE THERAPY

Extracorporeal shock wave therapy (ESWT) is an effective treatment for soft tissue and bone injuries that is readily accessible to most veterinarians. Indications include tendinitis, desmitis, osteoarthritis, and deep muscle pain.

The primary biological effects of ESWT include reduced levels of inflammatory mediators, increased levels of angiogenic cytokines resulting in vessel proliferation, increased levels of growth factors that result in tissue healing, increased numbers of osteoblasts, and recruitment of mesenchymal stem cells.[14,15] Pain relief has also been identified following shockwave treatment.[16]

Tissue compression and shear loads occur as the shock wave passes tissue interfaces, resulting in stimulation of bone and soft tissue healing.[17] ESWT treatment of arthritis of equine distal tarsal joints (bone spavin) resulted in improvement of lameness grade in 59 of 74 horses treated.[18] Chronic suspensory desmitis was successfully treated in 24 of 30 horses after 3 ESWT treatments.[19] ESWT is indicated for treatment of insertional desmopathy (such as at the origin or insertion of the suspensory ligament), dorsal cortical stress fractures, incomplete fractures of the proximal sesamoid bone, arthritis, and navicular disease and has also been used for treatment of tendonitis.

Treatment Protocols

For optimal outcomes, it is critical to have a specific diagnosis, accurate imaging that on follow-up will help determine treatment progress, and an appropriate rehabilitation exercise plan. Air blocks the sound energy of the ESWT device, similar to how poor transducer contact blocks transmission of sound energy during a diagnostic ultrasound examination. When treating heel pain through the frog, the site must be trimmed and placed in a wet bandage overnight. This wet bandage softens the frog and provides better penetration of the sound energy. For treatment of limbs and back, the treatment site is clipped and wiped clean of dust and dander. For certain anatomic regions, steps must be taken to allow optimal exposure of the target tissue to the energy impulse (**Fig. 6**). The horse is sedated in most circumstances.

Impulses
Small lesions, such as a collateral ligament of the distal interphalangeal joint, require 1000 impulses per treatment site. The most common suspensory desmitis lesions are administered 2000 impulses per treatment. Large areas of the back may require a total of 3000 impulses for each treatment.

Energy levels
- Soft tissue injuries less than 4 cm deep to the skin: 0.2 to 0.35 mJ/mm^2.[20]
- Soft tissue and bone in the heel region: 0.35 to 0.45 mJ/mm^2.[21] These levels are higher than the previous example because the penetration of energy is not as efficient.
- Backs disorders: 0.4 to 0.5 mJ/mm^2.[22] Higher levels are indicated because the deep muscle mass overlying the target tissues will absorb energy.
- Bucked shins and incomplete fractures: 0.35 to 0.55 mJ/mm^2.[23]
- Osteoarthritis: 0.15 to 0.3 mJ/mm^2.[24]
- Wounds: 0.1 to 0.15 mJ/mm^2.[25]

Focus depth
The focus point for ESWT should be the average depth of the lesion from the skin. Some ESWT devices use gel standoffs to focus the energy depth, and other devices use hand pieces with different focus depths.

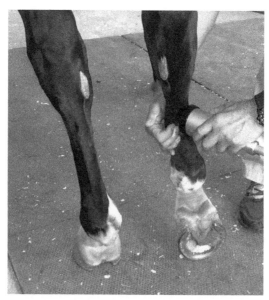

Fig. 6. The horse must be positioned with the fetlock flexed and the tendons displaced axially or abaxially for optimal energy exposure of the proximal suspensory ligament during extracorporeal shockwave therapy.

Aftercare and treatment intervals
The horse rests from exercise for 2 days following treatment. The horse then returns to the recommended rehabilitation exercise protocol. ESWT treatment is conducted at 2- to 3-week intervals for 3 sessions. The horse undergoes a full recheck examination 2 weeks following the third ESWT. At that examination, the decision is made to continue further ESWTs, to stop treatment, or to change treatment modalities.

LASER THERAPY

Indications for low-level laser therapy include wound therapy, treatment of soft tissue injuries, osteoarthritis, and local pain relief. The biological effects of laser include anti-inflammatory effects such as reduced IL-1 levels, reduction of pain sensation through reduced nerve depolarization and release of endorphins, and enhanced ATP production. The dose of energy required for treatment depends on the nature of the injury, depth of the tissue, and desired effect (stimulation of tissues for healing or anti-inflammatory and pain relief effects).[26]

There are a wide variety of laser devices available to the veterinarian. Wavelength and laser energy output are important considerations when choosing a device. Laser wavelengths for wound treatment should be in the 650-nm range, whereas treatment of deeper tissues requires wavelengths from 805 to 980 nm.[26] Lasers are available with energy outputs less than 500 mW and up to 15 W. Higher energy outputs reduce treatment time, but may cause undesired tissue effects if used incorrectly. Recommended laser dosage for soft tissue injuries is 4 to 12 J/cm^2.

A recent study by Haussler[27] found that laser combined with chiropractic therapy resulted in more pain relief for equine back pain than laser or chiropractic alone.

MANIPULATIVE THERAPY

Manipulative therapies such as stretching are methods of treatment that may be applied by the veterinarian and horse owner without the need for special equipment. Stretching is useful as a training aid to increase core strength; to maintain or increase neck, back, or limb joint range of motion; and for improving a horse's general flexibility. Specific issues that benefit from stretching exercise include neck or back pain, sacroiliac pain, and back muscle discomfort secondary to lameness.[7,28]

Range-of-motion exercises for the neck and back include so-called carrot stretches, whereby the horse is encouraged to bend the neck and trunk while reaching for a food reward. Use of such exercises has been shown to increase the cross-sectional area of the multifidus muscles that are primary stabilizers of the spine.[29]

The equine core muscles may be strengthened with work in side reins or long lines or using commercially available systems such as the Pessoa Training System (Dover Saddlery, Littleton, MA, USA) or Equiband (Equicore Concepts, East Lansing, MI, USA) training aids. The Pessoa system uses ropes and pulleys to adjust the horse's frame and neck position. A study reported that use of the Pessoa improved horse posture and stimulated core muscle activation.[30] The Equiband uses elastic bands around the trunk and hindlimbs to provide stimulation that engages the core muscle groups (**Fig. 7**).

Ground poles and cavaletti help activate a horse's full range of limb motion by strengthening the abdominal, back, and limb flexor musculature. This addition is very helpful to the rehabilitation exercise protocol because a horse returns to work and starts to develop strength. Comparisons of limb kinematics were made with poles set on the ground, at 11 cm and 20 cm above the ground. Hoof position was raised, and limb joint flexion was increased as ground poles were placed higher off the

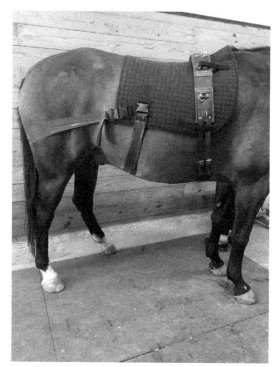

Fig. 7. This apparatus uses elastic bands around the trunk and hindlimbs to provide stimulation that engages the core muscle groups. The device may be used during in-hand work or while under saddle.

ground. The greatest amount of flexion and hoof raise was identified with poles placed 20 cm above the ground surface.[31] For strengthening during rehabilitation exercise or during early training, poles are initially placed on the ground at regular intervals (**Fig. 8**). The horse is walked or trotted over the poles. The height of the poles is increased as the horse develops strength and neuromuscular control. Ground poles set randomly may be used to improve proprioception and core balance (**Fig. 9**).[32]

EXERCISE

Exercise protocols are established during rehabilitation from injury or during return to work following a prolonged lay-up period. Controlled exercise is slowly increased depending on the level of conditioning or the injury status of the horse based on sequential ultrasound and lameness examinations. For most soft tissue injuries, hand walking should begin very soon after injury to encourage optimal fiber alignment and prevent restrictive adhesions. Exercise is started at the walk for 5 to 10 minutes once or twice daily (depending on lesion severity). Ultrasound and lameness evaluations should be repeated every 8 to 10 weeks, and exercise levels may be increased as parameters improve. According to Gillis,[33] controlled exercise alone resulted in successful outcomes for 67% to 71% of horses with soft tissue injuries. Pasture turnout resulted in successful outcomes in 25% to 51% of horses. An example of an exercise protocol applied for most soft tissue injuries is shown in **Table 2**.

All exercise must be adjusted for the level of soundness. If there is increased lameness, swelling is noted at the injury site, or if ultrasound parameters deteriorate, the

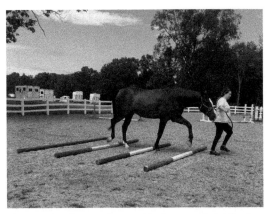

Fig. 8. Evenly spaced ground poles may be used to increase joint flexion and to re-establish eye-to-limb coordination.

exercise level must be decreased. Work at the trot should only begin after a solid 10 to 15 minutes hand walking for warm-up and should occur in short 1- to 1.5-minute segments.

Controlled exercise and exercise that minimizes concussion may be used during the rehabilitation period after injury or surgery. Exercise protocols have been established for rehabilitation of tendon and ligament injuries.[33] Gradually increasing the time and intensity level of exercise is beneficial for healing of soft tissues and bone because both tissues become stronger with use than with rest, particularly in growing horses.[34–36] Commonly, the horse is maintained in stall confinement with controlled exercise via hand walking, via ponying, or by use of a mechanical exerciser. Harness race horses may readily enter a controlled exercise program by designating the number of jogging miles at a given pace for each exercise session.

Ultimately, horses must work under the same conditions they will encounter in competition; this means that riding or driving with a gradual increase in duration and intensity of exercise will be needed. The key to retraining a horse is to realize that cardiovascular fitness declines significantly after 4 to 6 weeks of rest[37] and that

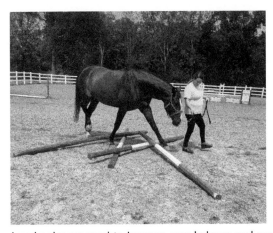

Fig. 9. Randomly placed poles are used to improve core balance and proprioception.

Table 2
Rehabilitation exercise protocol for equine soft tissue injuries

Weeks After Injury	Exercise	Confinement
0–4	5–10 min 2–3 times daily	Stall
5–8	10–15 min 3 times daily	Stall or small paddock
9–12	Increase time at the walk 5 min per week. Continue 3 times daily By 12 wk, good progress is walking 30–35 min each session	Stall or small paddock
13–16	If sound and continued improvement in lesion parameters: ride at the walk 20–25 min daily, hand walk 30 min daily	Stall or small paddock
17–20	Ride at the walk 30 min, add 3–5 min trot. On week 18, add 3–5 min additional trot per week	Stall or small paddock
21 to recovery	Ride at the walk 30 min, ride at the trot 15 min per session, add 3 min canter. On week 22–24, add 3–5 min canter per session	Small paddock

Adapted from Gillis CL. Rehabilitation of tendon and ligament injuries. Proc Am Assoc Equine Pract 1997;43:306–9.

bone strength decreases significantly within 12 weeks of rest.[38] Retraining will result in noticeable improvement of cardiac measurements within 6 weeks,[39] increased bone mineral density within 16 weeks,[40] and tendon dimensions within 16 weeks.[34] The studies on bone and tendon do not identify the earliest time that significant strength returns to these tissues so as to allow training or competition without reinjury. The author assumes that 3 to 4 months is the minimum time required to re-establish musculoskeletal tissue strength following a period of complete rest.

REFERENCES

1. Miklovitz SL. Thermal agents in rehabilitation. 2nd edition. Philadelphia: FA Davis; 1996.
2. Hayes KW, Hall KD. Manual for physical agents. In: Hayes KW, Hall KD, editors. 6th edition. Boston (MA): Pearson; 2012. p. 1–21.
3. van Eps AW, Leise BS, Watts M, et al. Digital hypothermia inhibits early lamellar inflammatory signaling in the oligofructose laminitis model. Equine Vet J 2012;44: 230–7.
4. Reesink HL, Divers TJ, Bookbinder LC, et al. Measurement of digital laminar and venous temperatures as a means of comparing three methods of topically applied cold treatment for digits of horses. Am J Vet Res 2012;73:860–6.
5. Kaneps AJ. Tissue response to hot and cold therapy in the metacarpal region of a horse. Proceed Am Assoc Eq Pract 2000;46:208–13.
6. Edner A, Lindberg LG, Broström H, et al. Does a magnetic blanket induce changes in muscular blood flow, skin temperature and muscular tension in horses? Equine Vet J 2015;47:302–7.
7. Denoix J-M, Pailloux J-P. Physical therapy and massage for the horse. 2nd edition. North Pomfret (VT): Trafalgar Square Publishing; 2001.
8. McGowan C, Goff L, Stubbs N, editors. Animal physiotherapy. Oxford (United Kingdom): Blackwell Publishing; 2007.
9. Levine D, Millis DL. Effects of 3.3 MHz ultrasound on caudal thigh muscle temperature in dogs. Vet Surg 2001;30:170.

10. Draper DO, Castel JC, Castel D. Rate of temperature increase in human muscle during 1 mHz and 3 mHz continuous ultrasound. J Orthop Sports Phys Ther 1995; 22:142–50.

11. Montgomery L, Elliott SB, Adair HS. Muscle and tendon heating rates with therapeutic ultrasound in horses. Vet Surg 2013;42:243–9.

12. Hayes BT, Merrick MA, Sandrey MA, et al. Three-MHz ultrasound heats deeper into the tissues than originally theorized. J Athl Train 2004;39:230–4.

13. Draper DO, Prentice WE. Therapeutic ultrasound. In: Prentice WE, editor. Therapeutic modalities in sports medicine. 5th edition. Madison (WI): McGraw-Hill; 2003. p. 103.

14. Notarnicola A, Moretti B. Biological effects of extracorporeal shockwave therapy on tendon tissue. Muscles Ligaments Tendons J 2012;2:33–7.

15. Caminoto EH, Alves AL, Amorim RL, et al. Ultrastructural and immunocytochemical evaluation of the effects of extracorporeal shock wave treatment in the hind limbs of horses with experimentally induced suspensory ligament desmitis. Am J Vet Res 2005;66:892–6.

16. Dahlberg JA, McClure SR, Evans RB, et al. Force platform evaluation of lameness severity following extracorporeal shock wave therapy in horses with unilateral forelimb lameness. J Am Vet Med Assoc 2006;229:100–3.

17. McClure S, VanSickle D, White R. Extracorporeal shock wave therapy: what is it? What does it do to equine bone? Proc Am Assoc Equine Pract 2000;46:197.

18. McCarroll GD, McClure S. Extracorporeal shock wave therapy for treatment of osteoarthritis of the tarsometatarsal and distal intertarsal joints of the horse. Proc Am Assoc Equine Pract 2000;46:200–2.

19. Boening KJ, Löffeld S, Weitkamp K, et al. Radial extracorporeal shock wave therapy for chronic insertion desmopathy of the proximal suspensory ligament. Proc Am Assoc Equine Pract 2000;46:203–7.

20. Lischer CJ, Ringer SK, Schnewlin M, et al. Treatment of chronic proximal suspensory desmitis in horses using focused electrohydraulic shockwave therapy. Schweiz Arch Tierheilkd 2006;148(10):561–8.

21. Turner TA. Diagnosis and management of palmar foot pain. Proc Am Assoc Equine Pract Focus Foot 2013;24–9.

22. Allen AK, Johns S, Hyman SS, et al. How to diagnose and treat back pain in the horse. Proc Am Assoc Equine Pract 2010;56:384–8.

23. Carpenter RS. How to treat dorsal metacarpal disease with tiludronate and extracorporeal shock wave therapies in thoroughbred horses. Proc Am Assoc Equine Pract 2012;58:546–9.

24. Frisbie DD, Kawcak CE, McIllwraith CW. Evaluation of the effect of extracorporeal shock wave treatment on experimentally induced osteoarthritis in middle carpal joints of horses. Am J Vet Res 2009;70(4):449–54.

25. Link LA, Koenig JB, Silveira A, et al. Effect of unfocused extracorporeal shock wave therapy on growth factor expression in wounds and intact skin of horses. Am J Vet Res 2013;2:324–32.

26. Hode L, Tunér J. Laser phototherapy. Grangesberg (Sweden): Prima Books; 2009.

27. Haussler K. Laser therapy. Proceedings, 8th International Symposium on Veterinary Rehabilitation and Physical Therapy. Corvallis, Oregon, August 3–8, 2014.

28. Stubbs NC, Clayton HM. Activate your horse's core: unmounted exercises for dynamic mobility and balance. Mason (MI): Sport Horse Publications; 2008.

29. Stubbs NC, Kaiser LJ, Hauptman J, et al. Dynamic mobilization exercises increase cross sectional area of musculus multifidus. Equine Vet J 2011;43: 522–9.

30. Walker VA, Dyson SJ, Murray RC. Effect of a Pessoa training aid on temporal, linear and angular variables of the working trot. Vet J 2013;198:404–11.
31. Brown S, Stubbs NC, Kaiser LJ, et al. Swing phase kinematics of horses trotting over poles. Equine Vet J 2015;47:107–12.
32. Paulekas R, Haussler K. Principles and practice of therapeutic exercise for horses. J Equine Vet Sci 2009;29:870–93.
33. Gillis CL. Rehabilitation of tendon and ligament injuries. Proc Am Assoc Equine Pract 1997;43:306–9.
34. Gillis CL, Meagher DM, Pool RR, et al. Ultrasonographically detected changes in equine superficial digital flexor tendons during the first months of race training. Am J Vet Res 1993;54:1797–802.
35. van Weeren PR. Exercise at young age may influence the final quality of equine musculoskeletal system. Proc Am Assoc Equine Pract 2000;46:29–35.
36. Reilly GC, Currey JD, Goodship AE. Exercise of young thoroughbred horses increases impact strength of the third metacarpal bone. J Orthop Res 1997;15:862–8.
37. Kriz NG, Rose RJ. Effect of detraining on cardiac dimensions and indices of cardiac function in horses. Proc Am Assoc Equine Pract 1996;42:96.
38. Porr CA, Kronfeld DS, Lawrence LA, et al. Deconditioning reduces mineral content of the third metacarpal bone in horses. J Anim Sci 1998;76:1875.
39. Shapiro LM, Smith RG. Effect of training on left ventricular structure and function. An echocardiographic study. Br Heart J 1983;50:534.
40. Firth EC, Goodship AE, Delahunta J, et al. Osteoinductive response in the dorsal aspect of the carpus of young thoroughbreds in training occurs within months. Equine Vet J Suppl 1999;30:552–4.

Index

Note: Page numbers of article titles are in **boldface** type.